NATURAL HEALING THERAPIES

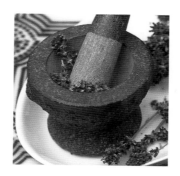

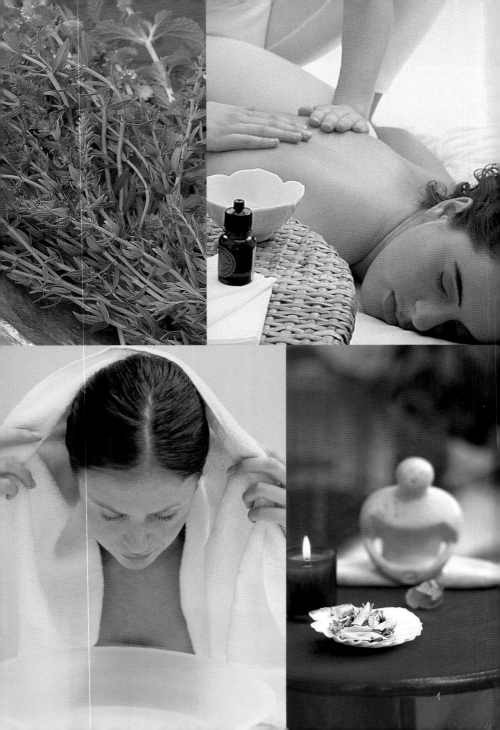

NATURAL HEALING THERAPIES

OVER 350 TIPS, TECHNIQUES AND
PROJECTS, SHOWN STEP-BY-STEP,
WITH OVER 800 PHOTOGRAPHS

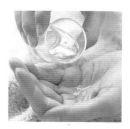

Raje Airey and Jessica Houdret

southwater

Southwater is an imprint of Anness Publishing Ltd Hermes House, 88–89 Blackfriars Road, London SE1 8HA; tel. 020 7401 2077; fax 020 7633 9499 www.southwaterbooks.com www.annesspublishing.com

UK agent: The Manning Partnership Ltd, 6 The Old Dairy, Melcombe Road, Bath BA2 3LR; tel. 01225 478444; fax 01225 478440; sales@manning-partnership.co.uk

UK distributor: Grantham Book Services Ltd, Isaac Newton Way, Alma Park Industrial Estate, Grantham, Lincs NG31 9SD; tel. 01476 541080; fax 01476 541061; orders@gbs.tbs-ltd.co.uk

North American agent/distributor: National Book Network, 4501 Forbes Boulevard, Suite 200, Lanham, MD 20706; tel. 301 459 3366; fax 301 429 5746; www.nbnbooks.com

Australian agent/distributor: Pan Macmillan Australia, Level 18, St Martins Tower, 31 Market St, Sydney, NSW 2000; tel. 1300 135 113; fax 1300 135 103; customer.service@macmillan.com.au

New Zealand agent/distributor: David Bateman Ltd, 30 Tarndale Grove, Off Bush Road, Albany, Auckland; tel. (09) 415 7664; fax (09) 415 8892

If you like the images in this book and would like to investigate using them for publishing, promotions or advertising, please visit our website www.practicalpictures.com for more information

Publisher: Joanna Lorenz
Editorial Director: Helen Sudell
Project Editors: Melanie Halton, Simona Hill and Catherine Stuart
Contributors: Raje Airey, Mark Evans, Jenni Fleetwood and Jessica Houdret
Designers: Jane Coney, Lilian Lindblom and Nigel Partridge
Production Controller: Pedro Nelson

Previously published as part of a larger volume, *The Handbook of Alternative Healing.*

10 9 8 7 6 5 4 3 2 1

Note

Contents

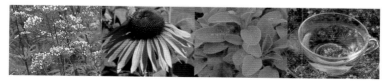

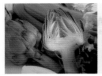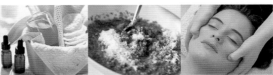

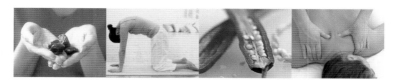

HEALING WITH AYURVEDA 256

AYURVEDA FOR COMMON AILMENTS 300

Introduction

Natural healing therapies aim to promote well-being by considering the unity between body, mind and spirit, and by harnessing the healing powers of organic ingredients. Many remedies in this book draw on ancient wisdom.

POWERFUL PLANTS

Flowers and herbs have formed the basis of medicine since the dawn of human history. Even today, it is estimated that about three-quarters of all conventional medicines are derived from living plants. However, plant remedies – that is, using plants in their natural state to heal ourselves, rather than their modern, manufactured drug counterparts – often mean that we can avoid many of the negative side-effects associated with conventional drug therapy (such as depleted nutrients, as well as unwelcome side-effects such as headaches, nausea and constipation).

The chapters on HEALING WITH FLOWERS and HERBS show how to grow, harvest, dry, prepare and store your own healing plants, and subsequently unleash their potent curative powers in floral and herbal teas, tisanes, infusions, inhalations and compresses. Treatments target specific ailments – such as chamomile

▼ SOME OF THE SIMPLEST HEALING METHODS REQUIRE US TO CORRECT MINOR HABITUAL ABUSES. YOU CAN AID YOUR DIGESTION, FOR EXAMPLE, BY RELAXING AS YOU EAT.

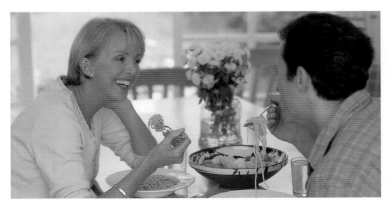

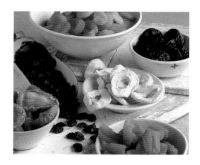

▲ RICH IN FIBRE, VITAMINS AND MINERALS, DRIED FRUITS MAKE GREAT HEALTHY SNACKS.

and cramp bark for an upset stomach, or rosemary tonic wine to relieve the winter blues. Each ailment has one or more healing recipes that are easy to make and simple to use. An alphabetical directory of the most effective healing plants offers further advice on the properties of each plant listed, with plenty of emphasis on how to use them safely. Always follow the guidelines given in the text and, if you are unsure as to the suitability of any remedy, call a qualified herbal practitioner for advice.

In HEALING WITH AROMATHERAPY the book eplores ways in which to use essential oils – the distilled essences of flowers, herbs, shrubs, vines, fruits, spices and trees – to lift the spirits, stimulate the senses, and even to alleviate conditions such as headaches, backache and premenstrual discomfort. You can add these potent oils to soothing baths and cleansing inhalations to benefit from their properties, or you may choose to use them in a restorative massage. There are also step-by-step instructions on how to perform the main massage strokes, as well as easy-to-follow massage routines for you to practise on a partner or baby, and self-massages for your own face, hands, arms and legs.

The natural perfume and protective properties of essential oils make them a perfect organic

▼ ADD ESSENTIAL OIL TO A NEUTRAL BASE TO MAKE A NATURAL SKIN CREAM.

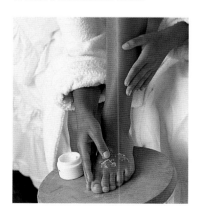

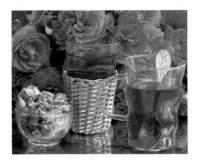

▲ HERBALISTS PRESCRIBE ROSE PETAL TEA TO PROVIDE COMFORT IN TIMES OF STRESS.

addition to luxurious skin creams, hair rinses and soaps, so there is plenty of practical advice on how to make these, too.

FORTIFYING FOODS

"You are what you eat" – never has this old adage seemed so appropriate. Scientific research is proving time and time again the therapeutic and preventative benefits of eating a nutritious variety of foods. For example, cruciferous vegetables (from the cabbage family), such as cabbage itself, as well as broccoli, water-cress and cauliflower, are rich in antioxidants, which are now known to help guard the body against cancer. By boosting our intake of these foods, as well as other antioxidant-rich foods, such as carrots, citrus fruits, tomatoes, and strawberries, we can help our body to entrap "free radicals" – unstable molecules that may attack perfectly healthy cells and cause illness. Furthermore, increasing our intake of the fatty acids that are present in oily fish and in nuts and seeds, supplies the body with a wide variety of benefits, ranging from healthy brain function to great-looking skin. This chapter explores these and other essential nutrients in our diet and shows just how easy it is to introduce them into our daily routine, with delicious recipes to help you get started.

Of course, it is not just what we eat that is important, but how we eat it. Taking each food-group in turn (fruits, vegetables, beans and so on), HEALING WITH FOOD provides a wealth of information on how to prepare and eat every kind of food for maximum nutritional benefit – whether learning simple ways to bring out flavour, eating wholewheat rather than processed-wheat products, or having your weekly vegetables delivered fresh from your local grower so that they have not had time to lose vital nutrients.

Brimming over with sumptuous suggestions for making healthy snacks, plus storage tips, advice on where to source essential vitamins and minerals (including an at-a-glance nutrient reference chart) and recipes for common ailments, HEALING WITH FOOD offers constructive and delicious advice on how to eat your way towards good health.

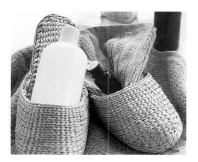

▲ TRY TO USE NATURAL FIBRES AND ORGANIC PRODUCTS AS OFTEN AS POSSIBLE.

ANCIENT HEALING

In the modern world we often view oursleves as separate from the world around us. However, the ancient practice of Ayurveda, which originated in India some 5,000 years ago, treats the self – meaning an individual's emotions, intellect, actions and physical

▼ A SOOTHING HEAD MASSAGE IS A WONDERFUL WAY TO RELIEVE A HEADACHE.

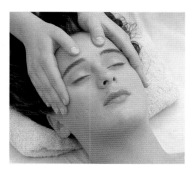

capacity – as being inextricably linked with the universe. HEALING WITH AYURVEDA offers practical ways to attune ourselves with the universal energies around us so that we can optimize our health and well-being. You'll learn about the Tridosha – the three universal energies – plus the ways in which to balance them, as well as about yoga and ayurvedic massage and aromatherapy. Complete a questionnaire on personality and physical traits to reveal your ayurvedic "dosha", or type, and use this knowledge to relieve illness and make lifestyle choices on diet, exercise, work and relaxation. In doing so, you will take your daily routine in a new direction that is entirely suited to you.

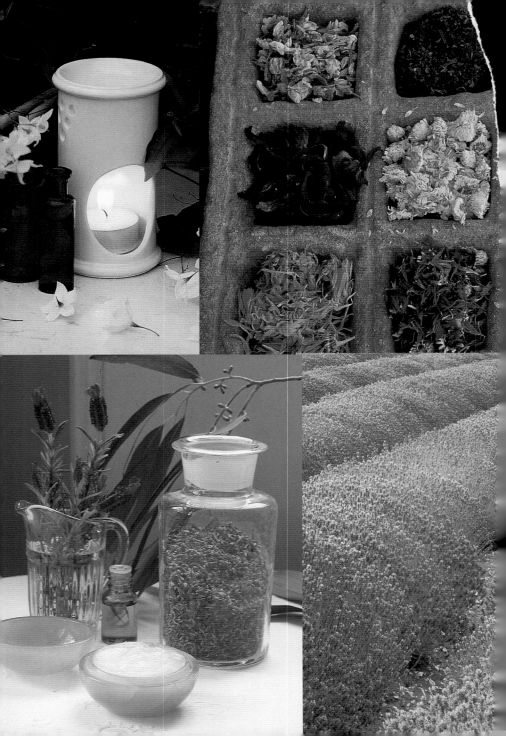

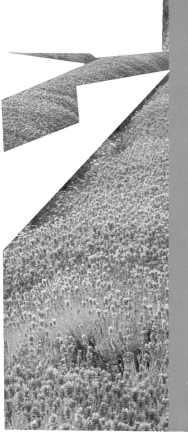

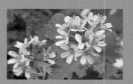

HEALING WITH
FLOWERS

Healing with flowers and herbs is as ancient as humankind, and, for much of our history, was the only medical option available. Even today, it is estimated that three-quarters of our pharmaceutical drugs are plant-based, and medical research continues to prove the healing powers of natural flower remedies.

The following section describes how to cultivate, harvest, dry, prepare and store healing flowers. It also explains how to use the various parts of a flower in therapeutic teas, tinctures, oils, infusions, compresses and inhalants. A directory of healing plants introduces some of the most useful flowers, with tips on how to recognize them and harness their healing properties.

History of healing with flowers

Until the advent of pharmaceutically based medicine at the beginning of the 19th century, healing systems in all cultures relied upon plants. Indeed, many of today's manufactured pills were originally made from plants.

EARLY HEALING SYSTEMS

Many ancient civilizations had well-developed medicinal plant healing systems. The earliest recorded natural healing methods were in China nearly 5,000 years ago, but because China remained closed to the West for many centuries, it is the texts recorded on tablets and papyri from the early civilizations of Sumeria and Egypt which are the antecedents of the later European healers. The great physicians of ancient Greece – Hippocrates, Galen, Theophrastus and Dioscorides – drew on these earlier cultures when writing their own works.

The name of Paracelsus (1493–1541), a 16th-century Swiss physician and alchemist, stands out in particular. He declared that he had not taken his knowledge from the Greek

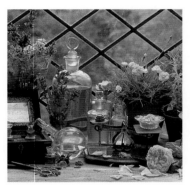

▲ FLOWERS HAVE BEEN USED FOR HEALING PURPOSES THROUGHOUT HISTORY.

"father of medicine" Hippocrates, the influential Roman physician Galen or anyone else, but "from the best teachers: experience and hard work". Paracelsus believed that disease originated from a departure with essential spirituality, and that by balancing the four elements, a substance called a "quintessence" was created, which healed the soul. The right essence, whether of a flower or mineral, would renew the connection with the spirit within, which was the true healer.

The renaissance

From earliest times there has been a belief in the power of flower fragrance to protect from disease. This led to the 15th-century production of pomanders, the use of posies, strewing herbs and herbal fumigation. Diet was also considered integral to healing – herbs and flowers were added to food for their medicinal action as much as for their nutritional or flavouring capabilities.

The modern era

In the early 19th century, the medical establishment moved away from remedies made with plants to laboratory-produced chemical drugs. This was a great step forward for civilization as general health improved and cures were found for many diseases, but a side-effect was that much of the responsibility for their own minor health problems was taken out of the hands of ordinary people and home remedies began to be forgotten.

During the last century Edward Bach (1886–1936), the founder of modern flower essence therapy, pioneered the treatment

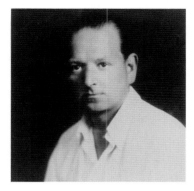

▲ Edward Bach, pioneer of modern flower remedies.

of the whole person by using safe and natural remedies. Of Welsh origin, Bach was born in Birmingham and trained as a bacteriologist. Later, in 1919, he joined the staff of the London Homeopathic Hospital.

Bach believed that for healing to succeed, the emotions, particularly fear, uncertainty and shock had to be addressed in depth. By 1928, he was experimenting with flowers, finding that impatiens, clematis and mimulus worked well to calm certain mental states.

Much ancient plant lore has recently been revived in the use of flowers in both internal and external forms of self-healing.

Using flowers to heal

The ways in which you can use flowers to heal include inhaling uplifting flower scents, drinking soothing teas, unwinding with a relaxing flower oil massage, or allowing the subtle energy of a flower essence to work on your deepest emotions.

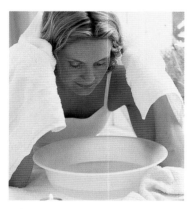

▲ AN ESSENTIAL OIL STEAM INHALATION
IS AN EXCELLENT WAY TO RELIEVE THE
CONGESTION OF A COLD OR BLOCKED SINUSES.

FLOWER OILS

Essential oils extracted from flowers have a powerful effect on mental and emotional states. Breathing in their vapours can be relaxing, restorative or uplifting. One way to inhale the scent is simply to put a few drops on a handkerchief and keep it on your pillow overnight. But for a more controlled and concentrated method, which is also longer lasting, an essential oil burner is ideal. Other ways of benefiting from oils include adding a few drops to a warm bath, or diluting and massaging into the skin.

FLOWER TEAS

Also known as tisanes, flower teas have been used for medicinal purposes for many centuries. Lavender, hyssop and thyme were taken to alleviate cold symptoms, while chamomile and lime flower were used against insomnia. Whatever the virtues, the scent of these tisanes alone is a tonic and they can be enjoyed simply for this reason.

FLOWER TONICS

Plants that affect the nervous system interact powerfully with the body. These are known as nervines, and invigorate and nourish the whole nervous system. Restorative nervine tonics include St John's wort, sage and mugwort. Relaxing tonics include skullcap, vervain and wood betony.

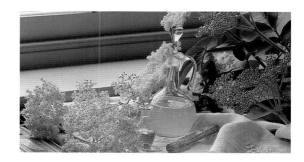

FLOWER ESSENCES

Natural flower remedies do not address the organs of our bodies, like our heart, liver and lungs, and their ailments. Rather, the remedies work on basic mental and emotional states.

Recent research suggests that water has a "memory" and can hold the imprint of a flower's properties, passing these on to us. Bach himself made sun-potentized flower essences in pure water.

Just as beautiful music can inspire us and help us feel whole, so can flower essences, Bach said. Some people now use the term "vibrational medicine" to make the analogy between music and the flowers clearer.

▶ THE SEPARATE COMPARTMENTS OF THIS SPECIALLY DESIGNED ESSENCE BOX KEEP THEIR INDIVIDUAL HEALING PROPERTIES CLEAR.

So, if our particular challenge is the anger or jealousy aspect of oversensitivity, holly essence will encourage acceptance of the emotion and bring out our love and tolerance. If the struggle is with the discouragement aspect of uncertainty, gentian essence can revive our courage and faith.

There is no harm in taking flower essences along with herbal tonics or essential oils, herb teas, aromas or inhalants. Each of these are healing expressions of the positive power of herbs and plants.

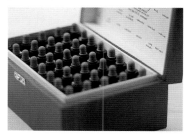

Flower cultivation

The process of cultivating, harvesting, drying and storing flowers can be a healing experience in itself. It is also the best way to learn the qualities of many remarkable healing plants, although buying flowers also gives good results.

GROWING

It is relatively easy to grow healing flowers, partly because many of these plants are wild in origin and do not suffer much from pests and diseases. Their aromatic smells often keep away harmful insects.

Cultivating your own healing flowers means you know exactly what has been put on them, and you can choose to go organic, using compost or mulches if you wish. Since many healing flowers are considered to be weeds — including red clover, horehound,

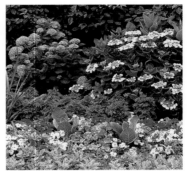

▲ MANY OF THE PLANTS FOUND IN GARDENS TODAY HAVE BEEN USED FOR THEIR HEALING PROPERTIES FOR 2,000 YEARS.

elder, selfheal and yarrow of those listed in the healing plants directory — they actually thrive on neglect and can colonize otherwise unused land.

HARVESTING

Reaping the flowers is a continuous rather than a one-off process. Most plants will be vigorous enough to allow repeated picking in small amounts, which encourages their further growth. It is best to gather flowers, stems and leaves when they are at their

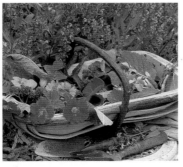

▲ GATHER FLOWERS IN THE MORNING, WHEN THE SUN HAS CAUSED THE DEW TO EVAPORATE AND ENCOURAGED THE FRAGRANCE TO DEVELOP.

peak, which for flowers means on a sunny morning and for leaves before flowering begins. Roots should be dug up in the autumn, cleaned and chopped into small pieces.

If gathering wild flowers, be sure you have identified the plant correctly. Use a wild flower book, and pick them away from busy roads. Many wild plants are protected by law and should be left alone.

DRYING

In order to dry flowers and herbs successfully, the moisture needs to be removed without losing the plant's volatile oils. Natural drying in an airing cupboard that is well ventilated is good. Loosely

▶ HANG BUNCHES OF FLOWERS UPSIDE DOWN TO DRY.

sealed brown paper bags can be used for drying small quantities. Using an oven even at a low setting is usually too hot for flowers and leaves, although it may be needed for roots.

STORING

Keep dried flowers and herbs in separate airtight containers in the dark, and label and date them. If hanging bundles, keep them in a dry, airy place out of the sunlight. If you prefer, store freshly gathered plants in the freezer. This method works well for lemon balm and parsley, which lose their flavour when dried. Tinctures are used to preserve selected herbs in alcohol.

BUYING

If buying flowers is your preference, choose ones that seem fresh, and which have retained their colour and aroma.

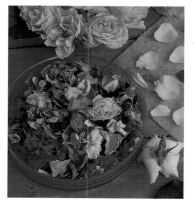

◀ DRIED ROSE PETALS MAKE A COLOURFUL AND FRAGRANT POTPOURRI WHICH CAN HELP TO PROMOTE A FEELING OF WELL-BEING.

Flower preparation

Flowers should be gathered on a warm dry morning, before the sun has become too strong and drawn out the essential oils. They are best picked in bud or freshly opened, when their scent and flavour are at their most enticing.

GATHERING FLOWERS

Those who are allergic to pollen should not eat flowers. In any case, it is still best to cut out the central reproductive areas, where the stamens and pollen are to be found, if you can. Individual flowers vary greatly but some, such as lilies and hibiscus, are particularly heavy with pollen and it is obvious which parts should be removed. With smaller flowers such as primroses, cowslips, violas and marjoram this would be difficult in the extreme, so if anyone is susceptible to allergy it is best to avoid all flowers.

Separate the petals from the green parts surrounding them – it is easier in some plants, such as marigolds, than others, for example violets or hollyhocks. Plants that flower in umbels, such as fennel, are best used whole.

▼ MAKE SURE THAT YOU IDENTIFY WILD FLOWERS CORRECTLY BEFORE PICKING THEM.

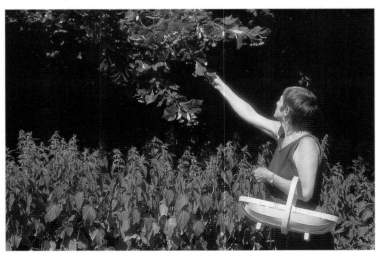

The body can benefit from the healing properties of flowers by using treatments both internally and externally.

INTERNAL USES

Flowers can be taken internally in infusions, inhalations, tinctures, teas, as capsules and powders, and in the many different types of preparations used to flavour and enhance cooking.

EXTERNAL USES

Flowers can be used externally in compresses, poultices, ointments, potpourris, skin creams, infused oils, massage and bath oils.

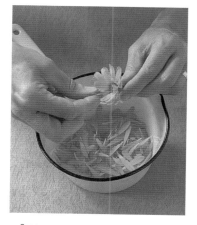

▲ CREAMS MADE FROM POT MARIGOLD PETALS ARE IDEAL FOR SOOTHING ALL MANNER OF SKIN IRRITATIONS.

▼ DRINKING SOOTHING HERBAL TEAS IS A GENTLE WAY TO RELAX BOTH BODY AND MIND.

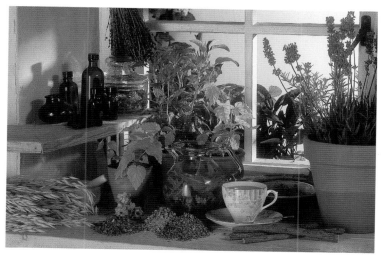

Infused oils and syrups

Active flower ingredients can be extracted in oil and used externally as a massage oil or added to creams and ointments. The two methods of extraction are hot infusion, using simmering heat, and cold infusion, using sunlight.

INFUSED OILS

Hot infusion is preferred for spicy herbs, including ginger or cayenne, and leafy herbs, such as comfrey, chickweed or mullein. The cold method is often used for fresh plants with delicate flowers, such as St John's wort, marigold, chamomile and melilot.

MAKING COLD INFUSED OILS

Pack a glass storage jar with the flowers or leaves of the herb. Pour in a light vegetable oil to cover the herbs, close the jar and shake well. Sunflower and grape

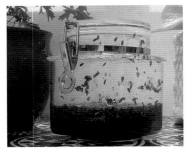

▲ PLACE THE FLOWERS AND THE OIL IN A GLASS JAR AND ALLOW THE CONTENTS TO STEEP FOR ONE MONTH IN A SUNNY LOCATION.

seed oil are good but olive oil is probably the best oil since it will not go rancid.

Allow the jar to stand on a sunny windowsill or in a greenhouse for a month, shaking it every day. The more sunlight there is and the longer the mixture is allowed to steep, the stronger it will be.

Strain the flowers or leaves, using a sieve or muslin bag. For a stronger infusion, renew the flowers in the oil every two weeks and infuse again. Pour the liquid into airtight bottles, label, and store in a cool dark place for up to a year.

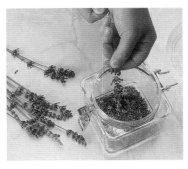

▲ FILL A GLASS STORAGE JAR WITH YOUR CHOSEN FLOWERS OR LEAVES.

Hot-syrup infusions

Since they use honey or unrefined sugar as a sweet preservative, syrups can disguise the taste of bitter plants such as motherwort or vervain. They are thus a good choice of remedy for children. Syrups are soothing in conditions such as sore throats and coughs.

Making syrups

Place 500g/1¼lb sugar or honey into a pan and add 1 litre/ 1¾ pints/4 cups water.

Heat gently and stir until the honey or sugar dissolves fully. Add 130g/4½oz flowers. Heat the ingredients gently for 5 minutes. Turn off the heat and allow the mixture to steep overnight.

Strain and store the syrup in an airtight container in the refrigerator or a cold cupboard. The sugar acts as a preservative so it should keep for up to 18 months.

▼ Keep prepared syrups and infused oils in airtight glass storage bottles in a cool dark place.

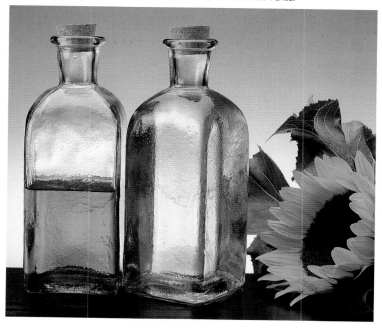

Flower essential oils

Aromatic flowers are so-called because they contain essential oils that carry specific and often therapeutic scents. The use of such oils and aromas to relax, sedate or stimulate has been known for millennia.

FLOWER THERAPY

Aromas have the power to produce emotional reactions within us. A distinctive smell can evoke a long-forgotten memory of a pleasurable or perhaps disturbing experience; it can be an instinctive reaction of attraction or repulsion, or a learned response. We quickly realize that hydrogen sulphide smells bad, like rotten eggs, while a rose is sweet. Some essential oils such as chamomile and lavender are sedating, others such as rosemary and geranium uplifting, but such general qualities can also be modified by our moods.

WHAT ARE ESSENTIAL OILS?
These are natural, volatile substances, which possess medicinal properties and a distinctive aroma. Essential oils evaporate easily, releasing their scent into the air, as demonstrated when someone brushes against an aromatic plant.

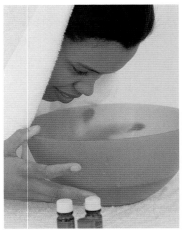

▲ STEAM INHALATION IS A QUICK AND EASY WAY TO ABSORB ESSENTIAL OILS.

Aromatherapy largely grew out of the perfumery industry, at first with the distillation of essential oils and later with the blending of aromatic oils to yield pleasurable scents. Combining oils is important to aromatherapy, as the effects of individual oils can be magnified in combination. A balanced scent from a blend is likely to be more enjoyable and have a greater therapeutic effect.

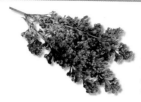

◀ AROMATIC PLANTS CONTAIN ESSENTIAL OILS THAT CAN BE USED TO RELAX, SEDATE, REFRESH OR STIMULATE.

In the early 20th century, the French chemist René-Maurice Gattefosse was working in the family perfumery laboratory, when he badly burned his hand. Plunging it into the nearest liquid, Gattefosse found that the jar of lavender oil he had accidentally used eased the pain, prevented scarring and promoted healing.

Gattefosse then began to examine the therapeutic properties of essential oils, and in 1928 coined the term "aromatherapy" to describe the use of aromatic oils for treating physical and emotional problems.

MASSAGE WITH ESSENTIAL OILS

Essential oils are very concentrated and can damage the skin. Before using them in massage, dilute them with a vegetable carrier oil, such as wheatgerm or almond oil. In general, mix one drop of essential oil with 10ml/ 2 tsp of carrier oil, but use less essential oil if there is any sign of a reaction.

Once diluted, essential oils have a short life, so prepare fresh mixtures in small quantities as needed. Use dry, clean utensils, measuring out about 10ml/2 tsp of vegetable oil into a blending bowl and adding the essential oil one drop at a time. Mix gently.

Body massage is a skill that takes some experience and knowledge of physiology, but essential oils can easily be self-administered for conditions such as chest colds or painful joints. Massage the spot gently with the diluted oils, then rest.

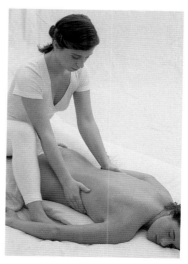

▲ THE NURTURING TOUCH OF MASSAGE IS ENHANCED BY THE AROMA OF ESSENTIAL OILS.

Flower essences

Although people have known of the medicinal benefits of flowers for centuries, modern flower essence therapy began with the work of Edward Bach in 1928. Flower essences are easy-to-use liquid herbal preparations.

A HOLISTIC APPROACH

As people's awareness and healing methods become more holistic, the flower essence philosophy of restoring our health by non-invasive treatment of mental-emotional conditions is gaining ground.

The essences are chosen according to how a person feels about their difficulty, a treatment process that is non-invasive. The compactness of the Bach set makes it a good starting point for people who are beginning their journey into flower essences.

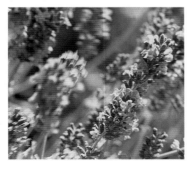

▲ "FLOWERS ARE CONSCIOUS, INTELLIGENT FORCES. THEY HAVE BEEN GIVEN TO US FOR OUR HAPPINESS AND HEALING." LILA DEVI

THE SEVEN HELPERS

Gorse	Heather
Oak	Olive
Rock Water	Vine
Wild Oat	

THE 38 BACH REMEDIES

The Seven Helpers are sun-potentized essences for deep, chronic conditions. They are used to support the Twelve Healers.

The Twelve Healers are sun-potentized essences, which correspond to the positive and negative states of 12 basic personality types. These "type essences" support us as we try to find balance and growth, and as we explore inner being throughout our lives.

The second half of the Bach 38 remedy set are essences prepared by the boiling method, and are known as the "New Nineteen Essences". These extend the work of the sun-potentized essences in developing positive spiritual qualities.

Negative	Essence	Positive
Restraint	Chicory	Love
Fear	Mimulus	Sympathy
Restlessness	Agrimony	Peace
Indecision	Scleranthus	Steadfastness
Indifference	Clematis	Gentleness
Weakness	Centaury	Strength
Doubt	Gentian	Understanding
Over-enthusiasm	Vervain	Tolerance
Ignorance	Cerato	Wisdom
Impatience	Impatiens	Forgiveness
Terror	Rock Rose	Courage
Grief	Water Violet	Joy

TRAVELLING SCENTS

Flower essences do "travel" quite well beyond their place of production, but some users insist on using essences prepared in their own country. In Australia, the bush essences are well known, while in the USA, Alaskan, Californian and Hawaiian essences are popular. In Europe there are French, Dutch and German essence makers, but the UK still has the largest number of makers and suppliers, including the Bach Centre in Sotwell and Findhorn and Harebell Remedies, Scotland.

THE NEW NINETEEN ESSENCES

Aspen	Elm	Mustard	Walnut
Beech	Holly	Pine	White Chestnut
Cherry Plum	Honeysuckle	Red Chestnut	Wild Rose
Chestnut Bud	Hornbeam	Star of Bethlehem	Willow
Crab Apple	Larch	Sweet Chestnut	

Nature's role in preparing essences

 Flower essences are prepared using either of two classical methods: sun potentizing or boiling. In both methods, flowers should be picked from plants growing in a clean, unspoiled environment.

THE DOCTRINE OF SIGNATURES

A belief popularized by Paracelsus nearly 500 years ago, is the doctrine of signatures. It holds that the appearance of a plant relates to its qualities and conveys a message to the healer.

Colour, shape, size and other features all offered insights to the flower healer. The dandelion's yellow colour, for example, suggested a role in healing liver complaints. The patches on lungwort leaves resemble diseased lungs, and the plant was used for bronchitis and tuberculosis.

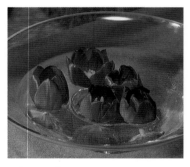

▲ A FLOWER'S ESSENCE ENTERS THE WATER.

This theory was very useful in the development of physical healing, while the Bach tradition has added the vital element of emotional healing.

THE "MEMORY" OF WATER

Edward Bach suggested in the 1930s that the sun is the catalyst which fuses water molecules with the imprint of the flowers used. His claims for potentization were supported by the French scientist Jacques Benveniste, whose experiments showed that water retains the imprint of a substance dissolved in it.

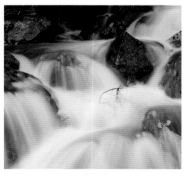

▲ WATER HAS THE POWER TO "MEMORIZE" THE IMPRINT OF FLOWERS.

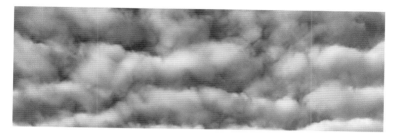

▲ IF CLOUDS APPEAR DURING THE SUN-POTENTIZING PROCESS, CONSIDER STARTING AGAIN ON ANOTHER DAY.

SUN-POTENTIZING METHOD

Start early in the morning. Fill a thin glass bowl with pure water. Pick your chosen flowers and float them on the water.

Leave the bowl close to where the flowers were growing, in clear sunshine for up to four hours or until the petals fade. The life force of the flowers will pass into the water, which may have changed colour, acquired flavour and feel "zingy" if held. Remove the flowers.

Pour the essence into a clean, clearly labelled bottle. Add an equal amount of brandy. This tincture now forms the "mother essence", which is diluted later to produce the dosage essence.

▶ FLOAT YOUR FRESHLY PICKED FLOWERS IN A BOWL OF PURE WATER FOR UP TO 4 HOURS.

BOILING METHOD

This is used for flowering trees, such as walnut, which need fire energy to bring out their essence, especially when the blooms are in spring, before the sun is hot.

Instead of picking only blossoms, add twigs too. Place the ingredients in a pan and cover with pure water. Bring to the boil and simmer for 30 minutes. When cool, filter the essence into a bottle with an equal amount of brandy. This tincture is diluted to create flower essence "stock", which can then be diluted for individual use.

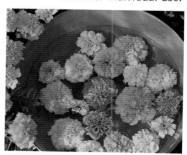

Using flower essences internally

Flower essences can be taken internally at any time of day, using a small dropper bottle. A few drops are taken several times a day, depending on the chosen brand, and treatment can be fitted easily into the daily routine.

TAKING ESSENCES

The best times to take the essences are morning and night, when the system is clear, and also before meals. A rhythmical approach like this will give the best results. No advantage is gained by taking a double dose if the previous dose has been forgotten, as taking more than the suggested number of drops is a waste.

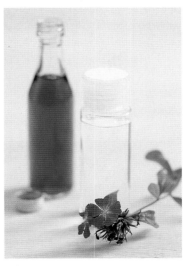

▲ STILL SPRING WATER AND BRANDY FORM THE LIQUID BASE IN DOSAGE BOTTLES.

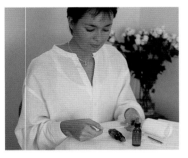

CLEARLY LABEL EACH DOSAGE BOTTLE WITH THE DATE AND CONTENTS LIST.

PREPARING A DOSAGE BOTTLE

1 Almost fill a 30ml/1fl oz dropper bottle with spring water. Add 5ml/1tsp brandy or vodka as a preservative. Use cider vinegar or glycerine if you prefer to avoid alcohol. For babies and animals, omit the preservative, but keep the bottle in the fridge.

2 Add 2 drops of each of your chosen mother essences to the water and brandy mixture. Bang the bottle on your palm to mix.

3 Carry the bottle with you, or prepare several dropper bottles of the essence and have these to hand for different situations.

Dosage is usually 4 drops, four times a day for 3 weeks. Then stop and allow a week to assess the results and decide what to put in a new bottle. Each treatment is based on a four-week cycle.

Alternatively, you may prefer to take essences internally by diluting in a glass of water, adding 2 drops per glass and stirring well. Sip four times a day, and make a fresh batch daily.

The essences can also be taken in pill form. To make the pills, weigh 25g/1oz sugar or lactose pilules in a small jar, add 2 drops of each chosen essence and shake well. Dry the pills on a plate. Chew two a day, with water.

There is no limit on the number of essences that can be taken together. Some herbalists like to use combinations of ten essences, while others will address a core issue using only one essence. Four essences in a treatment bottle is probably a good guideline.

▼ ONCE THE DROPS ARE DISPERSED IN A LARGE GLASS OF WATER, IT IS VIRTUALLY IMPOSSIBLE TO TASTE THE BRANDY.

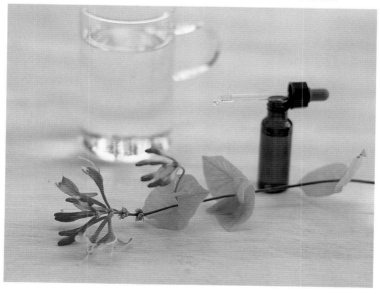

Using flower essences externally

The wide use of flower essences in oils and creams confirms their powerful effect when used externally. Many therapists believe that such usage greatly enhances the effect of the flowers.

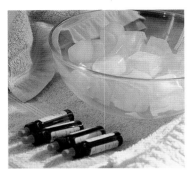

▲ ADD ICE TO A FLOWER COMPRESS TO EASE ACHES CAUSED BY SPRAINS AND SWELLINGS.

SOOTHING COMPRESSES

Lay the compress on any sprain, burn, bite or swelling, and repeat until relief is felt. Seek medical help if appropriate. Fill a bowl with hot or cold water, adding four drops of each chosen essence and four drops of essential oil. Soak a flannel or cotton wool in the water and apply to the affected area.

RELAXING ESSENCE BATHS

Add 12–20 drops of your current dosage essence in a warm bath, or four drops of each chosen mother essence, and swirl the water in a figure of eight pattern to activate the essences. Soak in the bath for 20 minutes and then rest for a further 20 minutes.

HEALING CREAMS

Use a hypoallergenic, non-perfumed cream as a base. Fill a jar with 50g/2oz cream, add four drops of each chosen essence and four drops of an essential oil. Mix with a wooden stick, screw on the jar lid. Apply the finished cream twice daily or as needed.

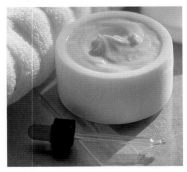

▲ ADD A FEW DROPS OF ESSENTIAL OIL TO YOUR FLOWER ESSENCE CREAM TO ENHANCE ITS HEALING PROPERTIES.

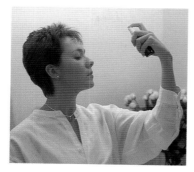

▲ USE FLOWER ESSENCE SPRAYS TO REFRESH YOUR MIND AND UPLIFT YOUR SPIRITS.

FLOWER ESSENCE SPRAYS

Sprays help to cleanse a room of negative energy and refresh stale air. Adding essential oils to flower essences gives an uplifting smell and heightens the healing benefits. Lighter oils such as lavender, geranium and lemon grass work best. Fill a plastic or glass spray bottle with 50ml/2fl oz spring water. Add 10 drops of essential oil and four drops of each chosen flower essence. Shake the bottle and spray as needed.

FLOWER ESSENCE MASSAGES

Put four drops of an essential oil and four drops of chosen flower essences into a bottle. Pour in 50ml/2fl oz of cold-pressed almond oil. Shake the bottle to mix and pour the contents into a bowl.

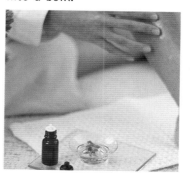

▲ ADD FLOWER ESSENCE TO MASSAGE OILS.

A FLOWER ESSENCE MASSAGE MIXTURE

- dandelion, for relaxing muscles
- comfrey, also to relax muscles
- chamomile, to relax involuntary muscle spasms
- rock water, to relax the whole body
- valerian, to release stress and tension
- orange hawkweed, to release trauma and energy blocks

Emergency essences

Most people's first introduction to flower essence therapy, and the most well-known of the Bach remedies, is Rescue Remedy. This emergency formula has proved to be helpful for all kinds of stressful situations.

RESCUE REMEDIES

The five classic components in Rescue Remedy are:

- rock rose, for fear
- impatiens, for mental agitation and tension
- cherry plum, for panic and fear of losing control
- clematis, for "faraway" feelings, and unwillingness to face up to a crisis
- star of Bethlehem, for treating panic and shock

Other composite remedies have names such as Five Flower Formula, Emergency Essence, Recovery Remedy, and Calming Essence. All work to restore our emotional and mental balance after shock or trauma, and in "heavy" situations, such as accidents, arguments, bad news, stress at work, or bereavement.

In a crisis, take four drops in a glass of water, sipping slowly. If no water is available,

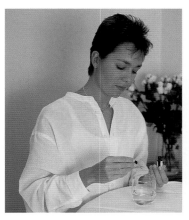

▲ IN A CRISIS ADD FOUR DROPS OF RESCUE REMEDY TO WATER.

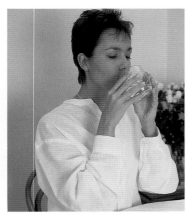

▲ THE QUANTITY OF WATER IS NOT IMPORTANT, BUT SIP SLOWLY.

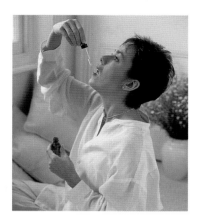

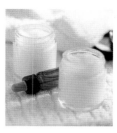
take directly on the tongue. Take the remedy every few minutes, as the effect is cumulative.

If a crisis is approaching, make up a dosage bottle: add four drops of Rescue Remedy to a 30ml/1fl oz dropper bottle of spring water. Add 5ml/1 tsp brandy and shake well. Take four times a day or up to 10 times if in need.

Carry a bottle of emergency essence with you at all times, and keep a bottle in the family first aid kit and in the office.

EMERGENCY SPRAYS AND CREAMS

The remedy can also be used as a spray or in cream form. To prepare the cream, add 10 drops of the remedy to 50g/2oz of a hypoallergenic base cream and mix. Useful healing additions are up to four drops of lavender or tea tree essential oil.

The cream should be applied at once if bruises, stings, cuts or blisters occur. Apply every two minutes or so for 15 minutes, as the skin absorbs the cream quickly. The liquid remedy should also be taken, or if no cream is to hand, the liquid can even be applied direct to the injury.

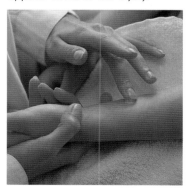

▲ APPLY CREAM IMMEDIATELY IF POSSIBLE.

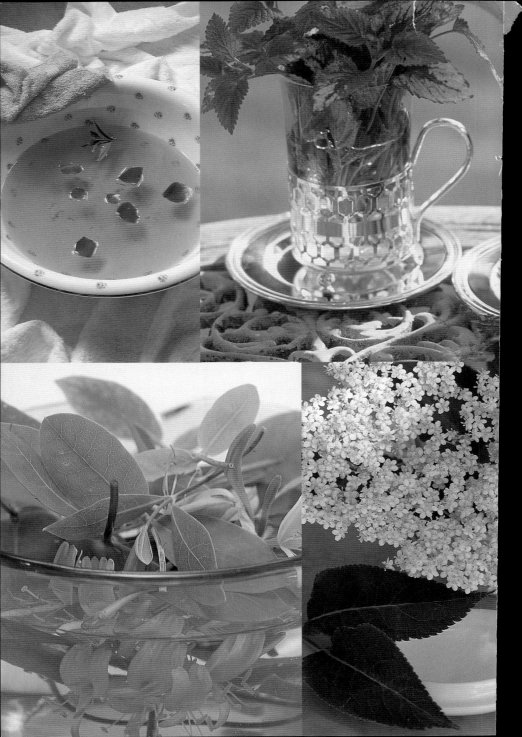

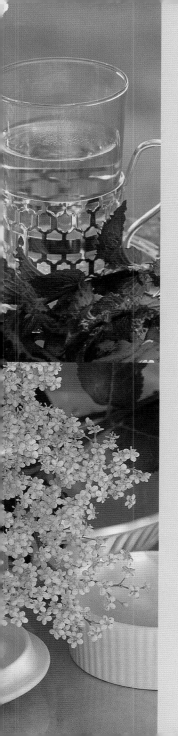

FLOWER
TREATMENTS

The flower remedies introduced in the following section will help you to deal with some of the difficult situations that we all experience from time to time. The recipes are designed to treat some of the most common health problems, from calming anxiety to relieving a painful abscess.

These natural treatments, which include the use of flower essential oils and essences, can be safely self-administered in the home, but do not exceed the doses stated, and seek further advice if you are pregnant or over 70 years of age. You can refer to the healing plants directory for further information, but always be sure to seek professional help if a problem persists or if you are uncertain.

Calming anxiety

Anxiety often involves over-excitement and frustration. In such states the body produces adrenaline but in the office or in traffic there is no safe outlet for all this negative energy. Flower remedies can help to calm you down.

ALLEVIATING SYMPTOMS OF ANXIETY
Flower essences and herbal treatments can help tackle symptoms of anxiety such as palpitations, sweating, irritability and sleeplessness.

Use Rescue Remedy in emergencies. If you can, take a hot bath, add lavender essential

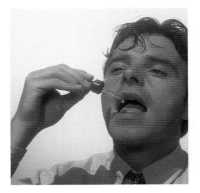

▲ TAKE A FEW DROPS OF RESCUE REMEDY WHEN SUFFERING FROM PANIC ATTACKS.

oil and relax. Passionflower, cut and dried when fruiting, is a good sedative and can relieve nervous conditions such as palpitations.

A TEA FOR ANXIETY
Try combining the nerve tonics and specific remedies listed. Put 5ml/1 tsp of three plants in a tea pot (use only 2.5ml/½ tsp passion flower). Add 600ml/ 1 pint/2½ cups boiling water, leave to steep for 10 minutes. Strain and drink. Take two cups a day for up to 2 weeks.

REMEDIES FOR ANXIETY
- To help calm your nervous system choose: oats; vervain; skullcap; or wood betony. These are all nervine tonics. Choose whichever one suits you best and combine it with a specific remedy for the symptom that troubles you most. Caution: these are powerful herbs, do not exceed the recommended doses (not more than 5ml/1 tsp a day of skullcap and betony, or 2.5ml/½ tsp if in combination).
- To ease palpitations: motherwort or passionflower.
- To reduce sweating: valerian or motherwort.
- To help you sleep: passionflower or valerian.

Fighting nervous exhaustion

We are more susceptible to illness or depression when hard pressed at work or when we face heavy emotional demands. Drinking flower teas is a safe and cheap way to support our nervous systems when stressed.

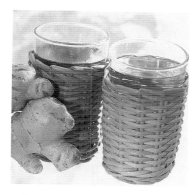

▲ A CUP OF GINGER TEA IS A TASTY TONIC FOR BOOSTING THE NERVOUS SYSTEM.

NERVOUS SYSTEM BOOSTERS

There are a number of flower and herb tonics that can strengthen the nervous system and prevent it running down to the point where nervous exhaustion occurs. Try ginseng, ginger, echinacea or hawthorn.

REVITALIZING TEAS

Mix equal amounts of the following six dried plants that work for nervous exhaustion: oats, licorice, skullcap, borage flowers, rosemary and wood betony.

Put 15 ml/1 tbsp of the mixture into a tea pot, and add 600ml/ 1 pint/2½ cups of boiling water. Steep for 10 minutes and strain. Take one to two cups daily for up to 2 weeks or until the exhaustion passes.

Vervain is another traditional healing plant with a reputation for restoring the nervous system following periods of tension. Vervain's aerial parts, including its stiff, thin stems and small lilac flowers, can be made into a bitter but stimulating tea. It has been used for centuries as an ideal tonic for convalescence from chronic illness.

A well-known restorative tea, for whenever you are tired or stressed, is Earl Grey, which acquires its distinctive flavour from the addition of bergamot oil. Note that the pure essential oil should not be taken internally.

▶ WOOD BETONY RESTORES THE NERVOUS SYSTEM.

Relieving PMS

Many plants have been found to have beneficial effects on the reproductive system, especially in women. Menstrual problems, including cramps, pre-menstrual syndrome and heavy bleeding, can be alleviated by self-treatment.

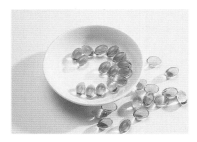

▲ CAPSULES OF EVENING PRIMROSE PROVIDE THE BODY WITH ESSENTIAL FATTY ACIDS, OFTEN LACKING WITH PMS.

Breast tenderness, sore nipples, and fluid retention can often accompany PMS. Lifestyle changes, such as eating extra fresh fruit and vegetables, stopping smoking, taking more exercise, cutting down on salt and processed foods, and relaxing by baths or meditation are all helpful in easing the symptoms.

Good remedies to try are evening primrose capsules or chaste tree (*Agnus castus*) tincture – 12 drops every morning for 3 months, are recommended. Vervain, valerian, lady's mantle and rosemary are also beneficial.

Vervain and rosemary are often taken in infusion form, while valerian is given as tablets or tincture. The name of lady's mantle refers to this plant's traditional value in healing women's conditions, especially in reducing heavy bleeding; it is best avoided during pregnancy.

VERVAIN AND LADY'S MANTLE TEA
Put 5ml/1 tsp each dried vervain and lady's mantle in a pot, and add 300ml/½ pint/1¼ cups boiling water. Steep for 10 minutes, strain and sweeten to taste. Take one cup twice a day from day 14 of the cycle, or from 2 weeks after your period begins.

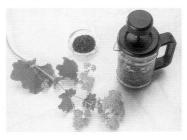

▲ LADY'S MANTLE AND VERVAIN TEA.

Easing periods

Pain during or before periods arises from contraction of the muscles of the womb, which reduces blood flow and causes the muscles to ache. Tisanes and hot compresses can help to ease these menstrual cramps.

Cramp bark (guelder rose) is well-known for reducing spasm, and rosemary is a circulatory stimulant and relaxant.

The leaves of feverfew, lady's mantle, peppermint and valerian have all been used in tisane form to relieve period pain. Among garden flowers, marigold petals in a tisane are known to normalize the menstrual process, and pasque flowers (use only the dried form in tisanes) are a noted relaxant. In each case, infuse 5–10ml/1–2 tsp of the leaves or flowers for up to 10 minutes in boiling water.

A hot-water bottle on the abdomen gives relief, as does a soothing hot herbal compress.

▲ ROSEMARY STIMULATES CIRCULATION.

HOT COMPRESS

Boil 10ml/2 tsp cramp bark in 600ml/1 pint/2½ cups water for 10–15 minutes. Add 10ml/2 tsp dried rosemary. Steep for 15 minutes and strain into a bowl.

Soak a clean cotton cloth or bandage in the liquid. When cool, wring out the cloth. Place the hot compress on the abdomen and relax until it cools.

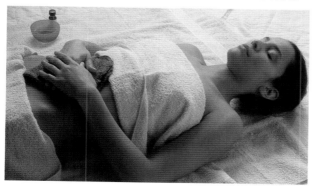

◄ PLACE A HOT COMPRESS ON YOUR ABDOMEN, LIE BACK AND RELAX.

Helping with the menopause

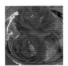

Menopause causes levels of the hormones progesterone and oestrogen to decline. This leads to reduced bone density and adds to the risk of osteoporosis. It is therefore important to support both hormones at this time.

Hormonal changes often lead to unpleasant hot flushes and night sweats. Using plant parts like the berries of chaste tree (*Agnus castus*), lime blossom and sage leaves will help maintain hormone levels, but general vitalizers or tonics are also useful in pepping up a run-down system.

Drinking rose water made by immersing damask rose petals in distilled water is a traditional remedy in the Middle East for alleviating the worst of menopausal symptoms.

TEA FOR HOT FLUSHES

Put 5ml/1 tsp each of motherwort flowers and sage leaves into a cup. Pour on 600ml/1 pint/ 2½ cups of boiling water. Sweeten with licorice (unless you have high blood pressure). Allow to cool, and sip throughout the day.

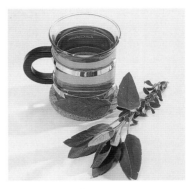

▲ TAKING REGULAR SIPS OF MOTHERWORT AND SAGE TEA THROUGHOUT THE DAY MAY HELP TO EASE MENOPAUSAL HOT FLUSHES.

LIME BLOSSOM TEA

The flowers should be gathered immediately after flowering in midsummer. Collect on a dry day and leave them to dry slowly in the shade. Use as a tincture or make a tisane by mixing a cup of boiling water with 5ml/1 tsp blossom. Leave to steep for up to 10 minutes, then allow to cool. Drink a cup three times a day.

> ### CAUTION
> Sage is a powerful herb and should only be taken for up to 3 weeks at a time. Allow a break of at least a week before taking again.

Lifting depression

Prolonged conditions of stress, anxiety and tension can lead to depression. Physical and mental energy leach away, leaving us vulnerable and unable to recover our equilibrium. There are, however, natural means of helping ourselves.

If external circumstances don't seem to be changing, sometimes all we can do is hang on to our routine until we feel able to cope again. Try to avoid taking pharmaceutical drugs or stimulants at this time. Cooking food may be hard to manage, so this could be the opportunity to buy fresh fruit and vegetables. Keep busy, walk more or do some grounding exercises. Give yourself extra time to relax. Helping others even when we feel depressed is very healing. Flower essences such as mustard, sweet chestnut and gentian, can address our depression, and wild rose and gorse can be used for hopelessness and despair.

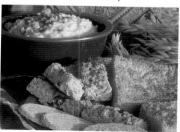

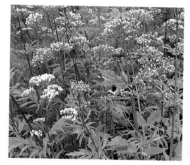

▲ THE ROOT OF WHITE-FLOWERED VALERIAN IS USED TO PROMOTE CALM AND SLEEP.

VALERIAN INFUSION

Use the dried and shredded root of valerian to make a remedy to calm the nerves. Using 10ml/ 2 tsp to a 250ml/8fl oz/1 cup of water, simmer the ingredients gently for 20 minutes in a covered, non-aluminium pan. Leave the concoction to cool, then strain. Re-heat and drink just before you go to bed to reduce the nervous tension and anxiety that hinder sleep.

◀ THERE ARE MANY TASTY WAYS IN WHICH YOU CAN INCREASE YOUR INTAKE OF OATS AS AN ANTIDOTE TO DEPRESSION.

Skin treatments

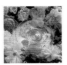

The skin needs regular cleansing and nourishment to remain healthy. Its condition reflects the general state of your body's health, but many minor skin problems can be improved by the external use of flower remedies.

ABSCESSES

A localized inflamed swelling containing pus is called an abscess. External abscesses on the skin can be treated with hot compresses, but internal abscesses in the mouth or other mucous membranes need qualified medical treatment.

To soothe an external abscess, make a compress by adding no more than 5–6 drops of an essential oil, such as bergamot, chamomile, lavender or tea tree, either separately or combined, to a bowl of boiling water and soak your compress in it. Keep this on the abscess for up to 30 minutes and renew when the compress cools.

ACNE

A common skin condition in adolescence, acne can affect people in later life

◀ WITCH HAZEL

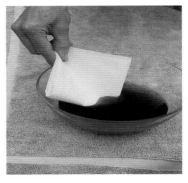

▲ USE A SOFT CLOTH TO MAKE A COMPRESS.

too. It is a sign that the sebaceous glands are producing excess sebum, and the glands and hair follicles are becoming blocked and infected.

Treat with the antiseptic and skin-growth-promoting essential oils tea tree, geranium, lavender or palmarosa, mixing a few drops into a bland carrier oil. Herbal treatments for external use include infusions of elderflower, lavender, marigold or witch hazel. Internally, a decoction of either red clover, burdock or echinacea can tone up the system.

Athlete's foot

This is a fungal infection that causes inflammation and itching between and under the toes, or in the groin. Preventive and controlling measures include scrupulously keeping the feet dry and clean, avoiding synthetic socks and tight-fitting shoes.

Use tea tree or lavender essential oil, or a clove of garlic, rubbed onto the skin twice or more a day. The Indian spice turmeric mixed with a tincture of marigold or myrrh can be applied between the toes.

Skin tonics

Stress and tension cause our muscles to contract, leaving the skin deprived of blood, and often resulting in dryness.

Make up a skin tonic by mixing essential oils into an unperfumed skin cream. Add either 3 drops rose and 3 drops sandalwood, or 4 drops neroli and 2 drops rose to a 25g/1oz pot of skin cream. Arnica, marigold, tea tree and witch hazel can also be applied in paste or cream form.

▸ Rose water is mild and soothing on the skin and also benefits the eyes.

A rose and chamomile facial

Hot water facials open up the pores and leave the skin refreshed and relaxed. Fill a wide bowl with hot water, add 3 drops rose and 4 drops chamomile essential oil. Cover your head with a towel and stay over the bowl for 5 minutes.

Relax for a further 15 minutes. Then apply a toning lotion: for dry skin, mix 75ml/5 tbsp rose water and 30ml/2 tbsp orange flower water; for oily skin, mix 90ml/6 tbsp rose water and 30ml/2 tbsp witch hazel.

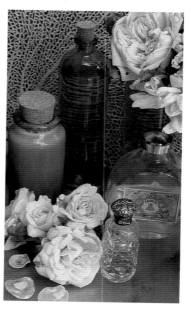

Respiratory ailments

The respiratory tract extends from inside the eyes and nose through the sinuses, throat and airways to the lungs. Flower treatments can combat infection, clear congestion, soothe the membranes and alleviate inflammation.

Avoidance of mucus-forming foods, such as dairy products and refined starches, is advised. So cut out morning cereals and milk, replacing with fruit or fruit juice. Also start taking raw garlic.

CATARRH

When the membranes of nose and throat are irritated, excess mucus may be formed, for example, after a cold. Nasal catarrh occurs higher up in the airways and bronchial catarrh lower down.

A steam inhalation of essential oils, with peppermint, alone or combined with eucalyptus, or tea tree oil helps to loosen mucus and fight infections. For longer-term catarrh, try oil of pine and lavender.

Infusions of peppermint or eucalyptus leaves or chamomile flowers help to ease nasal congestion, as can infusions of the herbs elderflower, golden rod and hyssop.

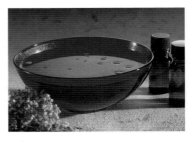

▲ STEAM INHALATIONS HELP TO CLEAR CONGESTION IN THE SINUSES AND CAN AID RECOVERY FROM COLDS AND SORE THROATS.

COLDS

It is difficult to stop a cold virus once it takes hold, and it will usually run its course. Flower treatments, though, can help to relieve symptoms and prevent catarrh or a worse infection taking over. Take plenty of fruit and vitamin C along with other treatments, and cut out mucus-forming foods.

Aromatherapy remedies include baths and steam inhalations. For night-time baths add 10 drops of lavender and 5 drops of cinnamon oil; earlier in the day, use tea tree or eucalyptus (10 drops of each).

A hot infusion of equal parts elderflower, peppermint and yarrow, taken before bedtime will raise the temperature and may sweat out the cold.

COUGHS

A cough is a reflex response to irritations or blockages in the airways, so it is better to help the cough rather than suppress it with drugs. Essential oils, such as lavender, thyme and eucalyptus, in a steam inhalation, will do this.

Among many good infusions are marshmallow, thyme, coltsfoot, echinacea and hyssop. For dry coughs, thyme and licorice are recommended, and for mucusy coughs, eucalyptus and licorice.

SINUSITIS

The sinus cavities are air spaces in the bones of the skull, around the eyes. Lined with mucous membranes, they are quickly infected by coughs or colds.

Steam inhalations using pine, peppermint, eucalyptus, tea tree, chamomile and lavender essential oils, singly or combined, are all

▶ AROMATIC PLANTS SUCH AS EUCALYPTUS ARE IDEAL FOR TREATING NASAL CONGESTION.

▶ PEPPERMINT

effective at loosening mucus. Catmint, elderflower and golden seal all make strong infusions.

SORE THROATS

A strong and effective treatment for sore throats and colds is a garlic, ginger and lemon mix: crush a clove of fresh garlic and a similar-sized piece of fresh ginger, adding the juice of a squeezed lemon. Add honey as a sweetener, and mix in hot water. Take up to three times a day.

Steam inhalations of oils such as lavender and thyme help to soothe a swollen throat, as will infusions or gargled tinctures of these herbs, or agrimony and sage.

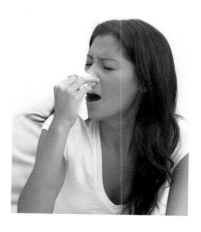

Digestive settlers

If we are what we eat, we owe it to ourselves to keep our digestive system in good health. The two main roles of plants and flowers in maintaining digestive peace are as stimulants and relaxants.

FOR STOMACH ACHE AND NAUSEA
A cramping stomach pain may be caused by poor digestion or food poisoning, nervous tension or infection. Stomach ache may lead to diarrhoea (see opposite). In general, marigold and garlic are good for fighting digestive infection, while relaxing herbs such as chamomile and cramp bark (guelder rose) will relieve stomach spasms. Nausea can be alleviated by taking frequent sips of a ginger infusion, or by diluting 10 drops of tincture in a glass of water. Lemon is a good cleanser.

FOR A NERVOUS STOMACH
You can make a soothing infusion from chamomile, lemon balm and hops, using them either together or separately.

⬧ MARIGOLD

Place 5ml/1 tsp each of chamomile flowers, peppermint and lemon balm into a small tea pot. Fill with boiling water and allow the tea to steep for 10 minutes before straining. Drink the tea three times a day or following meals. Hops can be added to the mixture in the evening to settle the stomach.

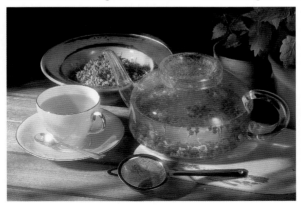

◀ CHAMOMILE TEA IS HIGHLY EFFECTIVE IN TREATING MANY DIGESTIVE DISORDERS AND FOR SETTLING THE STOMACH IN MOMENTS OF NERVOUS TENSION.

A SOOTHING COMPRESS

One of the easiest ways to settle an excited stomach is to use an aromatherapy compress, taking the time to relax and allow the soothing essential oils to ease your abdomen.

Measure out 2 drops orange and 3 drops peppermint or 3 drops chamomile and 2 drops orange into a bowl of hot water. Soak a flannel or a bandage in the mixture and place the compress onto the stomach. Lie back and relax for 10 minutes, or longer.

FOR WIND, BLOATING AND COLIC

Drinking hot teas of catmint, chamomile, ginger or peppermint will help to ease the symptoms. Alternatively, gently massage the abdomen in a clockwise direction with essential oils of chamomile, lemon verbena or peppermint. Dilute the oils at the ratio of 1 drop per 10ml/2 tsp of base oil.

FOR CONSTIPATION

One of the most effective methods of self-help is daily clockwise massage of the lower

▸ LEMON BALM MAKES A SOOTHING AND DELICIOUS TEA THAT CALMS THE STOMACH.

> ## CAUTION
> Hops are a sedative, so take only at night. Avoid licorice if you have high blood pressure, because it is high in sodium.

abdomen, and this can be performed using 2 drops of oils of lavender, marjoram or rosemary in 5ml/1 tsp of base oil. Alternatively, try chewing on a stick of licorice.

FOR DIARRHOEA

An infusion of agrimony or chamomile may help to reduce the impact of tension on the digestive tract. An infusion of meadowsweet may help to settle an acidic stomach. Thyme fights infections and improves digestion generally by settling churning, loose bowels and killing off harmful bacteria.

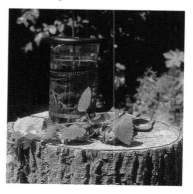

Enhancing sleep and relaxation

Flowers and herbs are unsurpassed in their ability to help us sleep and to relax. Sedative herbs aid in relaxation when taken at night, and stimulating herbs are used when we are overstimulated and there is nervous exhaustion.

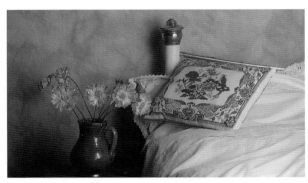

◀ A SOFT FLOWER PILLOW, WHETHER MADE OR BOUGHT, IS A GOOD FIRST STEP IN IMPROVING YOUR SLEEP ENVIRONMENT.

Sedative flowers often used in infusions are, in ascending order of strength, chamomile, lime, lavender and passion flower. Infusions in the evenings are relaxing, as are baths (see opposite). A hop or herbal pillow works for some people. The important thing is to take some time to relax and unwind, doing something peaceful after a day's work, such as gentle exercise, meditation, reading, yoga or tai chi.

SLEEPY-TIME TEA

Put 5ml/1 tsp each of dried chamomile, lemon balm and vervain in a pot, and pour on 600ml/ 1 pint/2½ cups boiling water. Steep for 10 minutes. Strain and drink a cup after supper and another before going to bed.

For a stronger blend, add a decoction of 5ml/1 tsp valerian root or 2.5ml/½ tsp dried hops or Californian poppy. Never take more than 2.5ml/½ tsp hops per day.

▼ CHAMOMILE TEA

Bath therapy

A hot bath, with the aroma of exotic flowers, and perhaps a candle and soothing music is an inexpensive, easily arranged yet unsurpassed relaxation therapy we can enjoy in our own homes.

In addition to quick baths or showers to get clean, we should often award ourselves the time for a relaxing bath, using essential oils to make our bathtimes particularly healing experiences. Pour 5 drops of an oil into the bath water just before you are ready to enter. This will form a thin film on the surface of the water, and the oil will be easily absorbed by the skin, whose pores are being opened up by the heat. Breathing in the aroma is also therapeutic for both the mind and body.

A refreshing morning bath is produced by adding 3 drops bergamot and 2 drops geranium oil. For an unwinding evening bath, blend 3 drops lavender and 2 drops ylang ylang. For aching muscles at any time, use 3 drops marjoram and 2 drops chamomile essential oils.

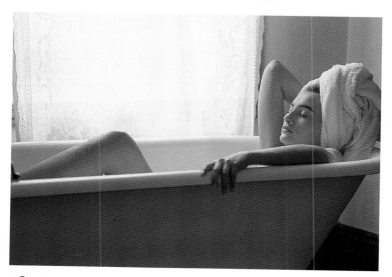

▲ TREAT YOURSELF TO A LONG BATH WITH ESSENTIAL OILS.

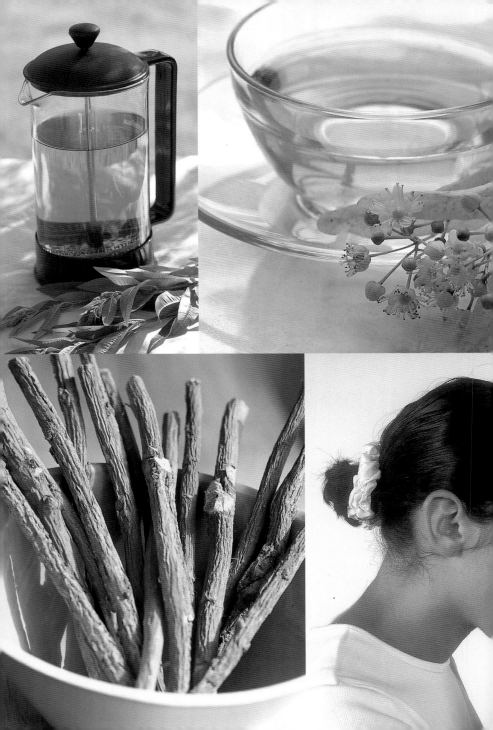

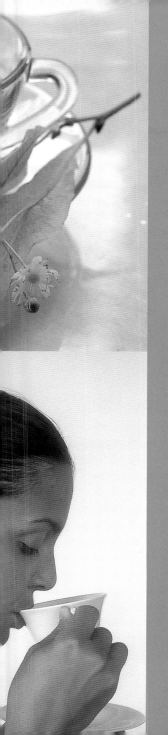

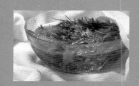

HEALING WITH
HERBS

Herbs have always played a key role in physical and emotional health, and many widely available herbs have a direct medicinal action, thanks to their antiseptic, antibacterial qualities. Cultivating healing herbs is easy – as shown in this section, they are prolific growers and require little effort in order to thrive. Taken as a regular part of the diet, sprinkled over food or used in a range of herbal teas and decoctions, herbs can help to ward off illness and cure minor ailments.

Other herbs have uplifting scents that promote a feeling of renewed energy when used externally in ointments, inhalations, essential oils, compresses and poultices. Refer to the healing plants directory for more information on the most useful herbs and their properties.

The benefits of herbs

The definition of what constitutes a herb has broadened over the centuries. Nowadays the term "herb" includes any plant whose roots, stem, leaves, flowers or fruit is used to flavour food, as medicine or for scent.

Most people are familiar with herbs that are commonly used in cooking, such as basil, bay, chives, mint, oregano, parsley, sage and thyme. But taking into account the broader definition of the term "herb", one can include plants such as aloe vera, spices such as ginger, flowers such as marigolds and roses, and fruits such as lemons and rose-hips.

As well as adding aroma and delicious flavour to food, culinary herbs have some nutritional value, often containing appreciable amounts of vitamins, minerals and trace elements. Adding herbs to your food on a daily basis actively promotes good health. Many herbs have excellent digestive qualities, helping the body to process and eliminate oily, fatty or gas-producing foods. But adding a generous sprinkling of fresh or dried herbs to your food is not the only way to benefit from these versatile plants.

▼ HERBS WILL GROW IN THE SMALLEST OF SPACES, SO LONG AS THEY ARE NURTURED.

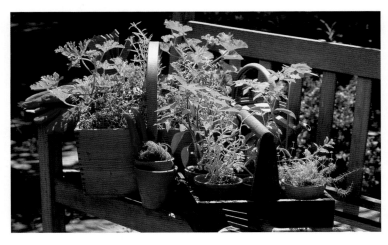

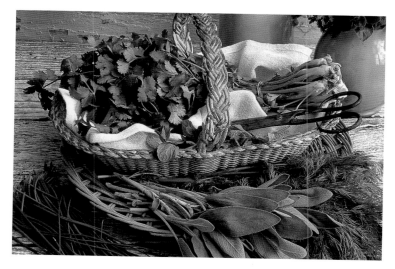

Herbal medicine

Many herbs have a therapeutic and medicinal value and can be taken in a variety of forms to prevent and cure illness and to promote health. Taken internally they can be made into herbal teas, decoctions, tinctures and inhalations. Externally they can be applied as compresses, poultices, ointments, creams or infused oils. Herbs add their aroma to bath water for a therapeutic soak and essential oils distilled from the flowers can be used for a massage.

Best of all, herbs are widely available and grow in the smallest of spaces ensuring a continual year-round supply for everyone.

▲ Fresh herbs aid digestion as well as adding vital flavour to food.

▼ Warming spices such as ginger and cinnamon add heat to food and drinks, helping to ward off colds and chills.

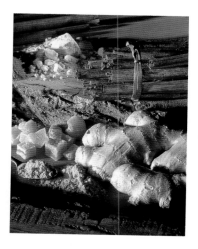

Growing herbs for healing

If you are new to growing herbs, take heart, they are not very difficult to grow and reward you over and over again for very little effort. The easiest way to start is to buy pot-grown herbs and plant them out.

SOIL

On the whole, herbs are undemanding and easy to grow. A free-draining lightish soil will suit the majority. Many herbs prefer light, sandy soils, similar to that provided by their Mediterranean homeland, and most will not stand heavy clay soils or waterlogged conditions. You can lighten soil by digging in sand, grit and organic matter, or you could consider growing your herbs in containers. The rule tends to be: silvery, needle-like leaves or tough foliage require sunny, well-drained conditions; soft green leaves tolerate partial shade; golden-leaved herbs will need sun.

▼ HERBS OFFER GLORIOUS SCENTS AND ADD STUNNING COLOUR TO A GARDEN.

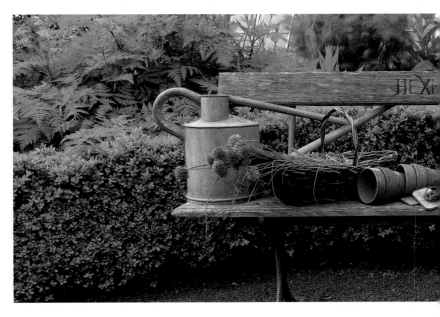

Site

A sunny, sheltered position protected from bitter winds will suit many herbs best. Some will need winter protection and a few, such as basil, will not survive and will need replanting every year. Aloe vera must be treated as a houseplant in colder regions.

Maintenance

Many herbs are prolific growers. Harvesting them helps to keep them under control, but do not be afraid to cut them back ruthlessly from time to time and root out those that are overpowering their neighbours. Herbs kept on a kitchen windowsill should be rotated with other container herbs to ensure that they do not become so bereft of foliage that they die.

Weeding

Remove weeds regularly to prevent them from competing with your herbs for moisture and nutrients. A light mulch of compost, applied in spring or autumn, can help to keep the herbs at their best.

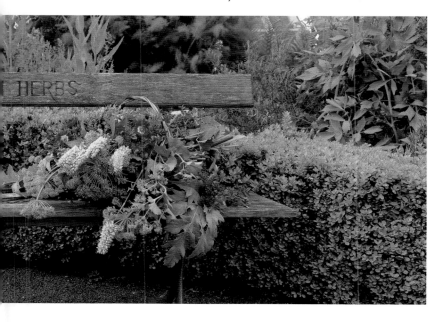

Growing herbs in containers

Herbs grow well in containers if you follow a few simple tips. Choose from a small pot, hanging basket, old clay sink, window box, large wooden tub or trough, old chimneystack or even an old barrel.

Make sure your container can give the roots room to spread out and that it has holes in the base. Put a layer of broken shards of terracotta pots in the base, then add a layer of sand or grit before filling with potting compost (soil mix). Never use garden soil, no matter what condition it is in – it may harbour weeds, pests and diseases. Add water-retaining gel if you like, since this helps with watering later on.

Extra fertilizer must be added after two weeks, with subsequent weekly feeds throughout the summer growing season to ensure you get the best from your plant.

Water frequently during the growing season. During the winter months water just enough to avoid drying out completely.

▼ A GROUP OF HERBS PLANTED IN DECORATIVE CONTAINERS CAN MAKE AN ATTRACTIVE FEATURE IN THE GARDEN.

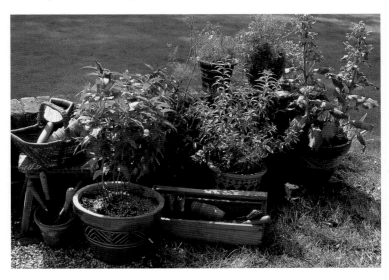

A trough for winter colds

Most of the herbs used here keep their leaves through the winter. However it is best to harvest them while they are growing vigorously and dry them for later use since they do not have the same potency while dormant in the winter.

You will need
  trough
  broken terracotta pots
  gravel or horticultural grit
  potting compost (soil mix)
  watering can

Herbs – black peppermint, hyssop,
  horehound, sage, purple sage,
  golden sage, thyme

▼ This trough will keep you supplied well throughout the year with herbs for teas and cough remedies.

1 Put a layer of broken terracotta at the bottom of the trough. Add a layer of gravel or horticultural grit. Almost fill with a good quality potting compost.

2 Tap the plants out of their pots and plant, firming around each one with extra compost. Put the tallest plants at the back and the thymes at the front. Top up with extra compost as necessary and water the plants in well.

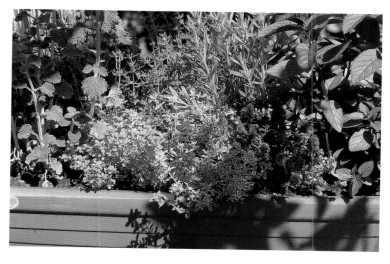

growing herbs in containers/a trough for winter colds **59**

Pots for headache remedies

Fresh or dried herbs made into teas and compresses can help to relieve the tension brought on by headaches and migraines. Feverfew will relieve a migraine, but it is bitter, so eat the leaves sandwiched between bread slices.

YOU WILL NEED

  half-barrel with drainage holes
  heavy-duty black plastic
  staples
  broken terracotta pots
  horticultural grit
  soilless compost (growing
    medium)
  sharp sand
  watering can

HERBS – feverfew, lavender, borage,
  marjoram, rosemary

▼ TAKING HERBS AS TEAS WILL HELP RELIEVE
THE SYMPTOMS OF A HEADACHE.

1 Insert the plastic liner into the tub and staple it to the side, overlapping the plastic where necessary.

2 Put in a layer of broken terracotta pots at the bottom, and top up with grit. Add soilless compost (growing medium), mixed with sand, to come a third of the way up the tub.

3 Fill with a gritty, open-textured potting compost (growing medium). Arrange the herbs in the tub. Plant up and water in well.

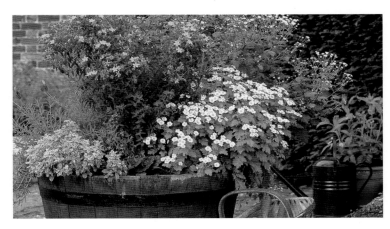

Pots for bites and bruises

The plants used here make good salves and ointments to counteract the effects of bites and bruises. If you are susceptible to bruising or live in areas infested with insects having herbs to hand will make life easier.

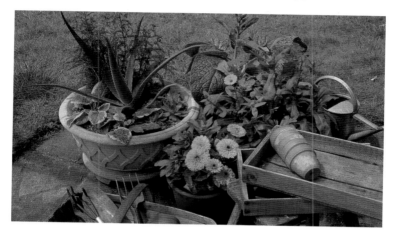

▲ HERBS WITH STRUCTURE MAKE STRIKING FEATURES IN POTS.

YOU WILL NEED
stone urn
broken terracotta pots
horticultural grit
loam-based potting compost
(soil mix) mixed in equal parts
with soilless potting compost
(growing medium)
trowel
watering can

HERBS – aloe vera, comfrey, house-leek, pot marigold, yarrow

1 Put a layer of broken terracotta pots in the base of the urn, then add a layer of grit.

2 Two-thirds fill the urn with the compost (soil mix).

3 Plant the aloe vera in the middle in its own pot so that it can be removed before the first frosts. Plant the yarrow and comfrey near the middle of the pot. Put the houseleeks around the outside, filling in with extra compost as necessary. Water the plants in well.

Harvesting herbs

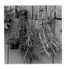 The best time to harvest the aerial parts of herbs is after their flower buds have formed but before they are in full bloom. Roots should be dug up in the autumn, cleaned and chopped into small pieces.

Never pick herbs without being able to correctly identify them, or pick so many that you reduce next year's growth.

Spread the herbs out to dry in an airy position out of direct sunlight – an airing cupboard is an ideal place. Leafy bunches can be tied into little bundles and hung up. Spread flower heads on tissue or newspaper and dry them flat. It can take a week for them to dry.

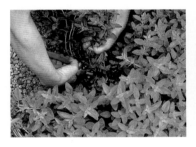

1 Cut bunches of healthy material at mid-morning on a dry day.

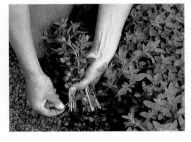

2 Strip off the lower leaves, which may otherwise become damaged.

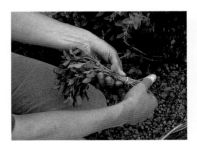

3 Bind the lower stems tightly with a rubber band.

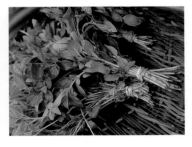

4 Gather as many bunches as you need, then hang them up to dry.

Storing herbs

The volatile oils in herbs start to deteriorate quickly once the herbs are put in the light. Store dried herbs in separate, airtight containers away from the light and they will keep for up to six months.

Although many herbs retain an aromatic scent for several years, for medicinal purposes it is best to replace stocks every year since their potency declines with age.

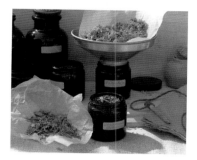

▲ DARK BOTTLES CAN BE USED TO STORE DRIED HERBS, OILS AND CREAMS.

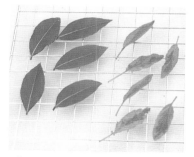

▲ DRY INDIVIDUAL LEAVES ON A WIRE RACK, BEFORE STORING THEM.

▼ SOME HERBS CAN BE LAYERED IN SALT TO PRESERVE THEM. THIS ALSO FLAVOURS SALT.

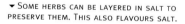
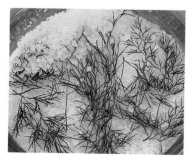

Many shops stock dried herbs. Buy these only if they seem fresh – brightly coloured and strongly aromatic. Some herbal remedies are now available over the counter in the form of capsules, tablets or tinctures. Choose the simpler types that tell you exactly the type and quantity of herb involved.

FREEZING HERBS

Instead of drying your herbs, you can store them in the freezer. This is especially useful for herbs such as parsley or lemon balm, which lose their flavour when dried.

Herbal teas

One of the easiest ways to benefit from the properties of a herb is to drink it as a tea. Taken regularly, herbal teas can make a significant contribution to well-being with their soothing, refreshing, and invigorating qualities.

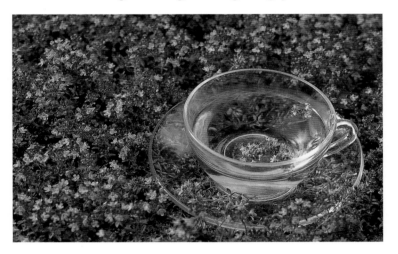

▲ THYME TEA IS GOOD FOR STOMACH CHILLS AND CHEST INFECTIONS.

Herbal infusions make wonderfully refreshing drinks and can be drunk as caffeine-free alternatives to ordinary tea and coffee. Herb teas, or tisanes, as they are sometimes known, are an acquired taste, so if you are unsure whether or not you like them, persist a little longer. The flavour of most can be sweetened with honey, a licorice stick, slices of fresh ginger or a squeeze of fresh lemon.

Herbal tisanes contain general health-giving properties and act as a refreshing tonic when taken regularly. Many commercial brands are available, but the taste is inferior to those made from fresh or

CAUTION

Herbs are powerful and can be harmful if taken in excess. Do not make teas stronger or drink them more frequently than recommended. Seek medical advice before taking herbal remedies when pregnant.

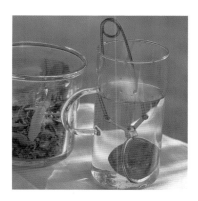

home-dried garden herbs. Using herbs from your garden also ensures that the maximum benefit will be extracted. Since many herbs have a specific medicinal quality, you could grow those that suit your needs for a year-round supply.

Herbal teas can be taken to help ward off colds and flu, to aid digestion, promote sleep, to relieve headaches, anxiety and stress, even to promote energy. Drink a cupful of the appropriate tea no more than three times a day. Teas can be stored for up to 24 hours in the refrigerator.

1 Allow either 30ml/2 tbsp fresh or 15ml/1 tbsp dried herbs to each 600ml/1 pint/2½ cups water. For a single cup (250ml/8fl oz), use two small sprigs of fresh or 5ml/1 tsp dried herb. Wash fresh herbs first.

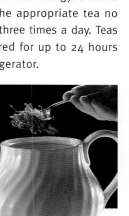

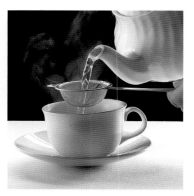

2 Put the herbs into a warmed pot. Pour on boiling water. Replace the lid to prevent vapour dissipation.

3 Leave to brew for three or four minutes, then strain the tea into a cup for a refreshing drink.

Herbal tea remedies

You don't necessarily have to feel ill to enjoy the benefits of a herbal brew, since many can be taken as a refreshing drink at any time of day. However, if you do have specific symptoms, the combinations below will certainly help.

Coughs and colds

PURPLE SAGE AND THYME	USE 5ML/1 TSP OF EACH FRESH PER CUP. ADD 1.5ML/ ¼ TSP CAYENNE PEPPER FOR A MORE POWERFUL EFFECT.
PEPPERMINT, ELDERFLOWER; CHAMOMILE AND LAVENDER	USE 2.5ML/½ TSP OF THE FIRST THREE, WITH A PINCH OF LAVENDER, PER CUPFUL OF WATER.
HOREHOUND	USE FRESH OR DRIED, AND SWEETEN WITH HONEY.
HYSSOP	USE FRESH OR DRIED, AND SWEETEN WITH HONEY OR MIX WITH ORANGE JUICE.
THYME	USE 5ML/1 TSP DRIED OR 10ML/2 TSP FRESH PER CUP.

Digestive troubles

CHAMOMILE	USE 5ML/1 TSP OF DRIED FLOWERS PER CUP.
PEPPERMINT AND LEMON BALM	USE FRESH HERBS IN EQUAL MEASURE AFTER A MEAL.
DILL	CAN BE GIVEN TO BABIES AND YOUNG CHILDREN. ALLOW 2.5ML/½ TSP LIGHTLY CRUSHED DILL SEED TO A CUP OF WATER AND BOIL FOR TEN MINUTES. STRAIN AND LEAVE TO COOL.
FENNEL SEED	CRUSH THE SEEDS AND SIMMER IN AN ENAMEL PAN FOR 10 MINUTES BEFORE STRAINING. CARAWAY SEEDS CAN BE PREPARED IN THE SAME WAY.
CINNAMON	INFUSE A CINNAMON STICK IN BOILING WATER FOR THREE OR FOUR MINUTES. LEAVE TO COOL, THEN CHILL.

Tonics and pick-me-ups

STINGING NETTLES	CHOP A SMALL HANDFUL OF YOUNG, FRESH LEAVES AND INFUSE IN 600ML/1 PINT/2½ CUPS BOILING WATER BEFORE STRAINING.
SPEARMINT	USE 15ML/1 TBSP CHOPPED FRESH LEAVES PER CUP AND SWEETEN TO TASTE.
GINGER	INFUSE FRESHLY GRATED ROOT GINGER IN TONIC WATER FOR A NATURAL ENERGY BOOST.

Early morning wakeners

LEMON VERBENA	USE FRESH OR DRIED LEAVES TO WAKE UP YOUR SYSTEM.
PEPPERMINT	USE ONE SPRIG OF FRESH HERBS PER CUPFUL.
BERGAMOT	USE FRESH FLOWERS FOR AN "EARL GREY" TASTE.

Disturbed sleep

CHAMOMILE	MAKE WITH 5ML/1 TSP DRIED CHAMOMILE TO A CUP AND ADD A PINCH OF LAVENDER FOR EXTRA RELAXATION.
LIMEFLOWER AND ELDERFLOWER	ADD A DASH OF GRATED NUTMEG AND SWEETEN WITH HONEY OR FLAVOUR WITH LEMON JUICE.
VALERIAN	USE 10ML/2 TSP DRIED AND SHREDDED ROOT TO A CUP OF WATER AND SIMMER FOR 20 MINUTES IN AN ENAMEL PAN WITH A LID. LET IT COOL, THEN STRAIN AND REHEAT IT.

Headaches, anxiety and depression

ROSEMARY	USE ONE OR TWO SMALL SPRIGS PER PERSON.
LEMON BALM	USE FRESH LEAVES.
BORAGE	USE FRESH OR DRIED FLOWERS.
PASSIONFLOWER, VALERIAN AND MOTHERWORT	USE 5ML/1 TSP DRIED VALERIAN AND MOTHERWORT AND ADD TO IT 2.5ML/½TSP OF PASSIONFLOWER.

▼ CHAMOMILE TEA IS SOOTHING AND CALMING.

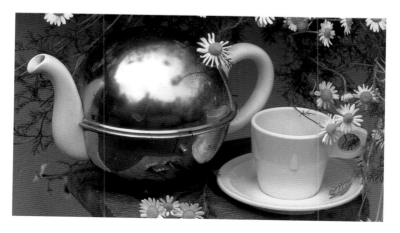

Herbal decoctions

Infusing herbs in boiling water is not enough to extract the constituents from roots or bark, such as valerian or licorice. Harder plant material needs to be boiled, and the resulting liquid is called a decoction.

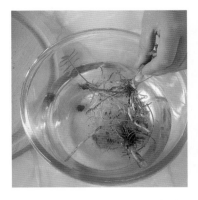

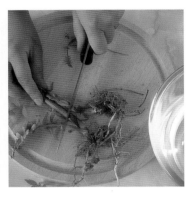

1 To make a decoction, wash the roots thoroughly.

2 Chop the root into small pieces.

3 Add 5ml/1 tsp of the root or bark to a pan of cold water. Leave it to soak for at least ten minutes, then bring it to the boil. Let it simmer for 10–15 minutes. Strain off the liquid and allow to cool before drinking. Decoctions can be kept for 24 hours in the refrigerator. They can be drunk hot or cold.

TIP
Always use a stainless-steel, glass or enamel pan when preparing herbal remedies.

Herbal decoction recipes

CHILBLAINS SIMMER 15G/½OZ CHOPPED GINGER ROOT IN 750ML/1¼PT/3 CUPS OF WATER UNTIL THE LIQUID REDUCES TO 600ML/ 1 PINT/2½ CUPS. STRAIN AND STORE IN THE REFRIGERATOR. TAKE 5–20ML/ 1–4 TSP THREE TIMES A DAY.

GALL BLADDER PROBLEMS SIMMER 50G/2OZ CLEAN, CHOPPED DANDELION ROOT IN WATER. STRAIN THROUGH A SIEVE AND STORE IN THE REFRIGERATOR FOR UP TO THREE DAYS. TAKE IN DOSES OF 5–20ML/1–4 TSP THREE TIMES A DAY.

Herbal tinctures

A tincture is a medicinal extract in a solution of alcohol and water. Take it diluted in a little water or fruit juice, but do not exceed 5ml/1 tsp, three or four times a day. Alternatively, use it externally, by adding it to liniments and compresses.

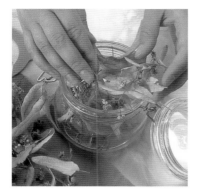

1 Place 115g/4oz dried herbs or 300g/11oz fresh herbs in a jar.

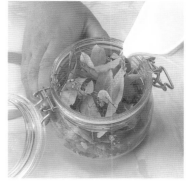

2 Add 250ml/8fl oz/1 cup vodka and 250ml/8fl oz/1 cup water.

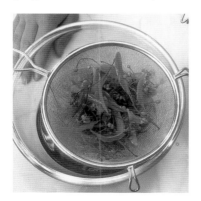

3 Leave to steep for two weeks, in a sunny place. Strain. Store in a dark, cool place for up to 18 months.

Herbal tincture remedies

HEADACHES AND DEPRESSION
USE LAVENDER IN THE QUANTITIES GIVEN ABOVE. TAKE DILUTED, OR ADD TO A COMPRESS.

MOUTH ULCERS AND INFLAMED GUMS
USE RASPBERRY LEAF IN THE QUANTITIES GIVEN ABOVE. DILUTE IN AN EQUAL QUANTITY OF WARM WATER AND USE AS A MOUTHWASH.

RHEUMATISM USE JUNIPER IN THE QUANTITIES GIVEN ABOVE AND ADD IT TO A LINIMENT FOR ACHING JOINTS.

COLDS AND HAYFEVER USE DRIED ELDERFLOWER IN THE QUANTITIES GIVEN.

Herbal ointments

 An ointment contains oils or fats, but not water, and helps to form a protective layer over the skin. For a natural method use a vegetable oil such as sweet almond or sunflower, with beeswax. This is easy to make at home.

BASIC RECIPE
25g/1oz beeswax
120ml/4fl oz/½ cup vegetable
  oil, such as almond, safflower,
  sesame, or grapeseed oil
  blended with almond oil.
20–30 drops essential oil, or
  10 drops if the ointment is
  for sensitive skin

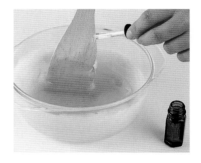

1 Place the beeswax and the oil in a glass bowl over a pan of water. Bring the water to the boil and simmer until the wax has melted into the oil. Remove from the heat.

2 Stir continually as the oil/wax mixture cools and stiffens. Add your choice of essential oils and stir into the mixture.

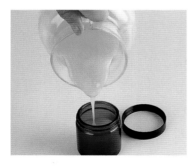

3 Pour or spoon into small, clean ointment jars, seal and store. Make small quantities and use it as soon as it is made.

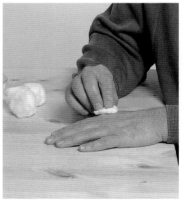

▲ APPLY OINTMENTS SPARINGLY AND COVER THE TREATED AREA TO PROTECT FROM DIRT.

Herbal creams

Making an organic cream is very similar to making an ointment, again using beeswax. Keep the cream in a cool place away from direct sunlight, and preferably in a dark glass or china pot. It should not be kept indefinitely.

BASIC RECIPE

25g/1oz beeswax
25ml/1½ tbsp water
120ml/4fl oz/½ cup vegetable oil such as almond, safflower, sesame or grapeseed oil
20–30 drops essential oil, or 10 drops if the ointment is for sensitive skin

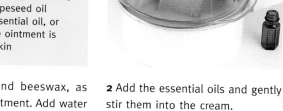

1 Melt the oil and beeswax, as for the herbal ointment. Add water to the melted wax/oil mixture, drop by drop, stirring all the time until the cream thickens and cools.

2 Add the essential oils and gently stir them into the cream.

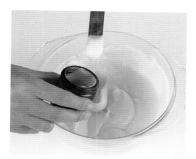

3 Carefully pour or spoon the cream into small, clean dark-coloured ointment jars. Seal and then store in the refrigerator.

Herbal cream recipes

PROBLEM SKIN ADD ROSE OIL.

MATURE SKIN ADD JASMINE OIL.

FOR HEALING CUTS AND GRAZES ADD MARIGOLD OIL.

FOR HEALING ACNE ADD SANDALWOOD OIL TO THE CREAM.

TO NOURISH, CLEANSE AND SOOTHE THE SKIN MELT 50G/2OZ WHITE BEESWAX WITH 115G/4OZ ALMOND OIL. IN A SEPARATE BOWL DISSOLVE 2.5ML/½TSP BORAX IN 50ML/2FL OZ/¼ CUP OF ROSEWATER. SLOWLY POUR THE BORAX MIXTURE INTO THE OIL AND WAX, WHISKING UNTIL IT COOLS. WHEN IT THICKENS POUR INTO GLASS POTS.

Herbal poultices

Mashed herbs form the basis of a poultice. Its main purpose is to aid the healing of bruises, sprains and sores. Poultices are applied direct to the skin, either hot or cold. Hot poultices help sprains, while cold help inflammations.

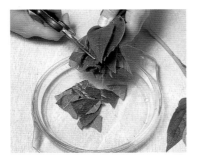

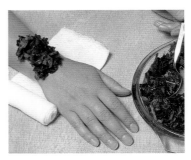

1 Snip a handful of herb leaves into a dish. Cover with boiling water and mash to a pulp with a spoon.

▾ A POULTICE IS AN INSTANT METHOD OF USING HERBS.

2 Leave to cool slightly, then spread the pulp directly on to the affected area. Cover with a piece of gauze and a bandage. Leave in place for several hours.

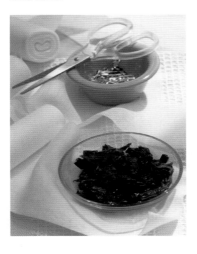

Herbal poultice recipes

SUNBURN LIGHTLY CRUSH THE LEAVES AND STEMS OF ANGELICA AND APPLY DIRECT TO THE SKIN.

GRAZES AND SCRAPES MASH SAGE LEAVES. APPLY DIRECT TO THE SKIN.

ACHING JOINTS AND MUSCLES MIX EQUAL AMOUNTS OF THE FRESH OR DRIED LEAVES OF MARJORAM AND ANGELICA AND APPLY TO THE SKIN.

STINGS AND BITES MIX OATMEAL TO A PASTE WITH AN INFUSION OF COMFREY OR MARIGOLD. LEAVE TO COOL. APPLY TO THE SKIN.

Herbal compresses

A compress is a length of fabric that is applied to the skin after it has been dipped into a herbal infusion. Compresses are gentle remedies that can be used for many different complaints from headaches to period pains.

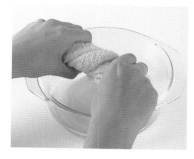

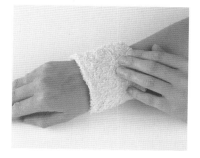

1 Put fresh or dried herbs into a clean bowl. Pour over boiling water. Leave to stand for one hour, then strain the liquid. Allow to cool and mix in any essential oil. Soak a length of cotton in the infusion and wring out lightly.

2 Position on the affected area and hold in place with a bandage.

▼ COMPRESSES CAN BE USED EFFECTIVELY ON ANY PART OF THE BODY.

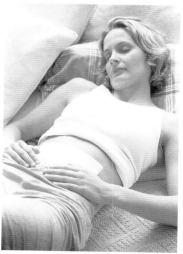

Herbal compress recipes

TIRED EYES USE A SMALL HANDFUL OF CHAMOMILE FLOWERS TO MAKE AN INFUSION. DIP MUSLIN IN THE COOLED LIQUID AND APPLY TO THE CLOSED EYELIDS FOR 20 MINUTES.

BRUISES MAKE AN INFUSION USING 25G/1OZ FRESH WORMWOOD OR 15G/ ½OZ DRIED WITH 500ML/17FL OZ/ 2¼ CUPS BOILING WATER. LEAVE FOR 30 MINUTES THEN STRAIN. APPLY COOL.

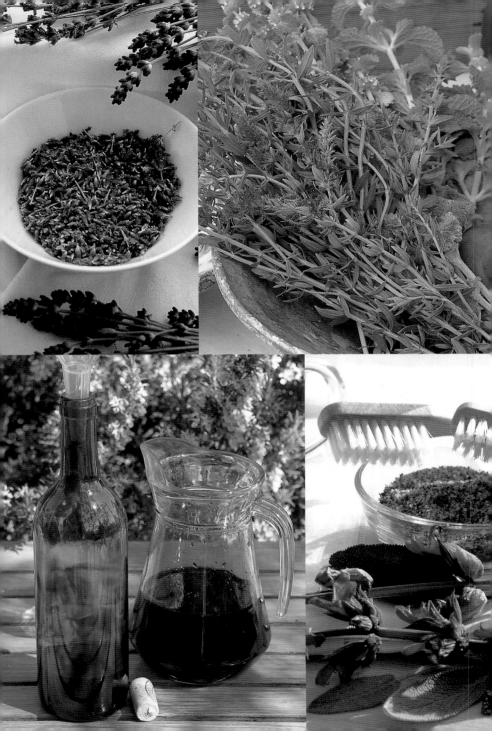

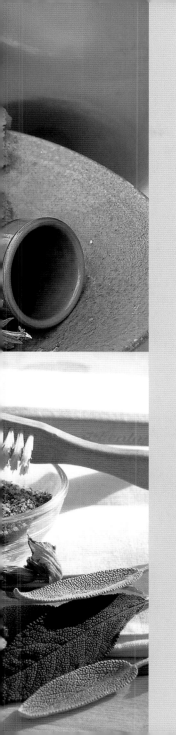

HERBAL
TREATMENTS

The recipes that follow use the roots, bark, leaves, stems and flowers of many kinds of herbs in healing remedies for everyday complaints such as cuts, bruises, aches and winter blues. Be aware that, while herbs are therapeutic if used in the correct quantity and manner, they are also a potent source of medicine, containing essential oils which can become toxic if dosage is exceeded.

Pregnant women should avoid any herbal remedies unless under professional supervision. Always use herbs from a reliable source, and if you are unsure of what the herb is, do not use it. Consult the healing plants directory for more information on key herbs and their properties, but always seek further advice if unsure.

Coughs and colds

The common cold affects most people at some point in the year. And since there are over 200 strains of cold virus, it is not surprising that a cure has not been found. Herbal treatments can help to relieve many of the symptoms.

GARLIC COLD AND FLU SYRUP
With antiseptic and antibacterial qualities, garlic is ideal for a cold.
INGREDIENTS

> *1 head garlic, crushed*
> *300ml/½ pint/1¼ cups water*
> *juice of ½ lemon*
> *30ml/2 tbsp honey*

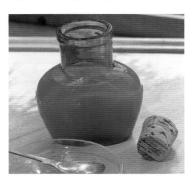

1 Bring the garlic and water to the boil. Simmer gently for 20 minutes.

2 Add the lemon juice and honey and simmer for two minutes. Allow to cool, then strain into a clean, dark bottle with an airtight lid. Take 10–15ml/2–3 tsp three times a day. Keep chilled for up to three weeks.

EVERYDAY ROSE-HIP TEA
Rose-hips are high in vitamin C and help to ward off colds.
INGREDIENTS – MAKES ABOUT 6 CUPS

> *45ml/3 tbsp rose-hips*
> *1.5 litres/2½ pints/6¼ cups*
> *filtered or bottled still water*

1 Top and tail the rose-hips. Cover them in tap water for 24 hours. Strain and discard the water.

2 Bring the filtered water to the boil. Add the rose-hips. Simmer for about 30 minutes. Strain and serve, sweetening to taste with honey.

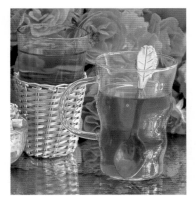

LAVENDER AND EUCALYPTUS VAPOUR
The fresh and uplifting scents of lavender and eucalyptus clear the bronchial and nasal passages. Rub on the chest before bedtime.

INGREDIENTS

50g/2oz petroleum jelly
15ml/1 tbsp dried lavender
6 drops eucalyptus essential oil
4 drops lavender essential oil

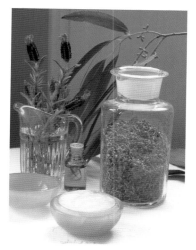

1 Melt the jelly in a bowl over a pan of simmering water. Stir in the lavender and heat for 30 minutes.

2 Strain the liquid through muslin. Cool, then add the oils. Pour into a clean jar and leave until set.

▲ THIS VAPOUR RUB CAN ALSO BE INHALED. MELT A SMALL QUANTITY IN A BOWL OF STEAMING WATER. LEAN OVER THE BOWL, WITH A TOWEL OVER YOUR HEAD AND INHALE. KEEP THE CREAM REFRIGERATED.

Herbal cough remedies

TRY A WARM INFUSION OF ONE OR A MIXTURE OF THE FOLLOWING:

COLTSFOOT – PARTICULARLY GOOD FOR IRRITATING, SPASMODIC COUGHS

HYSSOP – A CALMING AND RELAXING EXPECTORANT

MARSHMALLOW – FOR A HARSH, DRY, PAINFUL COUGH

THYME – POWERFULLY ANTISEPTIC, THIS RELIEVES A HARSH, DRY AND PAINFUL COUGH

HOREHOUND – AN EXPECTORANT, FREEING UP MUCUS AND HELPING IT TO BE REMOVED.

Herbal cold remedies

TAKE AN INFUSION OF EQUAL AMOUNTS OF PEPPERMINT, ELDERFLOWER AND YARROW JUST BEFORE BED TO INDUCE A SWEAT. YOU CAN ALSO ADD:

CAYENNE PEPPER – USE 1.5ML/¼ TSP OF THE POWDER TO STIMULATE THE SYSTEM. CAYENNE ADDS INSTANT HEAT AND WILL MAKE YOU SWEAT.

CINNAMON – BREAK A CINNAMON STICK INTO THE HERBS FOR A GENTLE, WARMING AND SWEAT-INDUCING EFFECT.

GINGER – GRATE A SMALL PIECE OF FRESH ROOT GINGER INTO THE MIXTURE FOR EXTRA HEAT.

Sore throats

Often a sore throat goes hand-in-hand with the symptoms of a cough or cold. Sometimes sore throats can be caused by air conditioning in office buildings. Discomfort can be eased by gargling with herbs or sipping herbal teas.

ALLIUM STEAM INHALATION

Garlic has antiseptic properties that will ease a sore throat.

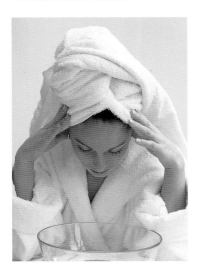

1 Put two unpeeled garlic cloves in a heatproof bowl containing 1 litre/ 1¾ pints/4 cups of steaming water.

2 Lean over the bowl, cover your head with a towel and inhale the garlic steam for several minutes.

▶ HYSSOP YIELDS BOTH FLOWERS AND LEAVES WITH MEDICINAL BENEFITS.

HYSSOP TISANE

Originally from Asia, hyssop is a widely-used medicinal plant with beautiful aquamarine flowers and aromatic leaves with expectorant properties. When used alone, it makes an excellent tisane for coughs and sore throats, but it is quite bitter, so it's worth adding a little honey, or a splash of orange juice for vitamin C, to sweeten the taste.

To prepare, simply infuse a few fresh or 5ml/1 tsp dried leaves and flowers in 250ml/8fl oz/1 cup boiling water.

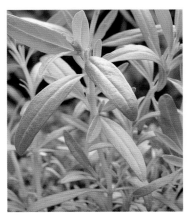

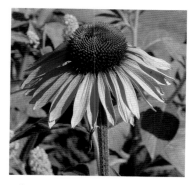

▲ THE CONEFLOWER, *ECHINACEA ANGUSTIFOLIA* OR *E. PURPUREA,* BOOSTS THE IMMUNE SYSTEM AND MAY BE TAKEN IN TABLET FORM OR AS A TINCTURE.

Soothing laryngitis

Laryngitis is an acute inflammation of the larynx or vocal chords, leading to a sore throat, hoarseness and even loss of voice. Local treatment is by gargle or cold infusions. The best herbs to use are sage, thyme, agrimony or raspberry leaf. Leave a small handful of leaves to infuse in boiling water, then strain and allow to cool. For a soothing effect, add marshmallow.

Tonsillitis remedies

MAKE AN INFUSION OF AGRIMONY, LICORICE, SAGE, OR THYME TO GARGLE WITH. A TINCTURE OF MYRRH IS ALSO GOOD.

Thyme and sage gargle

This recipe will relieve sore throats, mouth ulcers, gum disease, laryngitis and tonsillitis.

INGREDIENTS
> 15g/½oz fresh sage and thyme, or horehound
> 600ml/1 pint/2½ cups boiling water
> 30ml/2 tbsp cider vinegar
> 10ml/2 tsp honey
> 5ml/1 tsp cayenne pepper

1 Put your choice of herbs into a bowl, pour in the boiling water, cover and leave for 30 minutes. Strain the liquid.

2 Stir in the vinegar, honey and cayenne. Gargle or swallow 10ml/ 2 tsp at a time, twice a day.

▼ SAGE AND THYME ARE BOTH ANTISEPTIC.

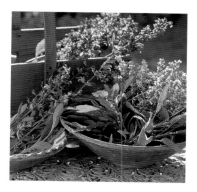

Blocked sinuses

Inhaling steam scented with aromatic herbs relieves the congestion of a cold or blocked sinuses, and can remove headaches which are often a symptom of the problem. You could put essential oils on your pillow and in your bath too.

ESSENTIAL OIL INHALANT

Add 5 drops of eucalyptus, 2 drops of camphor and 1 drop of citronella essential oils to 600ml/1 pint/ 2½ cups of boiling water and inhale.

FRESH HERB INHALANT

To relieve blocked sinuses, immerse fresh herbs and spices in steaming water and breathe in the vapours. Choose from: eucalyptus leaves, basil, cayenne pepper, cinnamon stick, hyssop, juniper berries and foliage, lavender, lemon balm, mint, rosemary, sage, thyme.

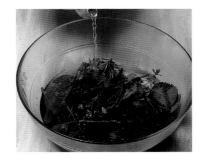

1 Put a large handful of your chosen herbs in a bowl and pour in about 1 litre/1¾ pints/4 cups of boiling water. Lean over the bowl, covering both it and your head with a towel. Inhale deeply.

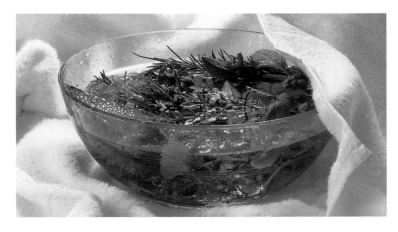

Earache

Earaches most often develop through an infection, often following a cold or sinusitis. They should not be neglected – infections can spread through into the middle or even inner ear with potentially serious complications.

If earache is associated with catarrh, this should be treated too. Earache in children needs to be treated quickly as an infection in the middle ear can be both painful and damaging. Seek medical help if earache worsens or persists.

Do not put anything into the ear, unless it has been examined by a doctor to check that the eardrum has not been perforated.

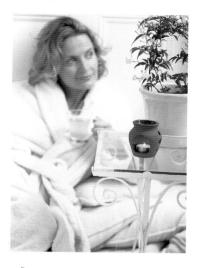

▲ Burning lavender and chamomile oil will bring relief to earache sufferers.

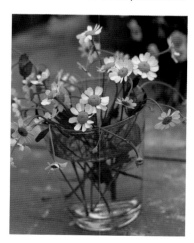

▲ Chamomile contains the anti-inflammatory chemical azulene which is useful for treating conditions such as earache, acne, insect bites and allergies.

Earache remedies

Chamomile – make a hot compress, or an infusion. Apply to the outside of the ear with cotton wool (swab).

Garlic – eaten with food, or if the eardrum is not perforated, crush 1 clove of garlic into 5ml/1 tsp of olive oil; warm it to blood temperature and gently insert a few drops into the ear. This is an excellent antibiotic.

Winter blues

The transition from autumn to winter is not always easy, particularly when the nights draw in and the warm weather disappears. To help you to adapt to this changing time, there are plenty of uplifting herbal remedies.

ROSEMARY TONIC WINE

This pungent and aromatic herb has a long tradition of use as a tonic herb with a reputation for lifting the spirits.

INGREDIENTS

handful of fresh rosemary
    leaves
2 small cinnamon sticks
5 cloves
5ml/1 tsp ground ginger
grating of nutmeg
bottle of claret or other good
    quality red wine

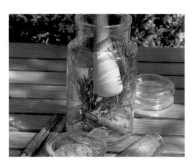

1 Put the rosemary, cinnamon and cloves into a jar and crush using a pestle to release their essential oils. Add the ginger and nutmeg to the mixture.

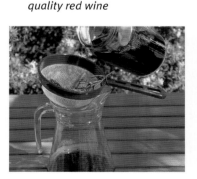

2 Add the wine, seal the jar and leave in a cool place for ten days. Strain into a sterilized bottle and seal with an airtight stopper.

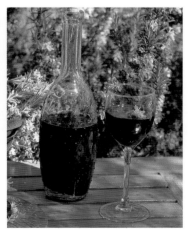

▸ GINGER TEA CAN BE ENJOYED AS A WINTER WARMER, OR IN SUMMER BY ADDING ICE.

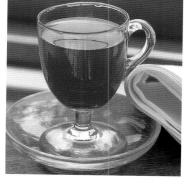

WINTER WARMER

Ginger is one of the oldest and most popular herbal medicines, and makes an excellent, warming addition to a cup of tea on a cold day. This uplifting drink helps to ward off low blood sugar, headaches, nausea and fatigue.

To make the tea, pour boiling water over a teaspoon of freshly grated ginger root. Add the juice of half a lemon and sweeten with 1 tsp of honey. Drink warm in winter as an uplifting tonic or allow to cool thoroughly, and add ice, for a deliciously chilled tea in summer.

▸ FRESH OR HOME-DRIED HERBS MAKE THE BEST HERBAL TEAS, BUT IF YOU DON'T HAVE ACCESS TO A SUPPLY, THERE ARE SOME GOOD SHOP-BOUGHT VARIETIES.

ALCOHOL-FREE TONIC

This excellent tonic should be drunk warm twice a day for a total of three weeks to thoroughly cleanse the system. Add 600ml/ 1 pint/2½ cups of boiling water to 2.5ml/½ tsp each of oats, vervain and borage. Flavour with peppermint or licorice. Allow to steep for ten minutes and strain.

AROMATIC BOOSTER

Pulsating with freshness and the promise of spring, this delicate infusion is perfect for reawakening the senses at a dark time of year. Simply add three or four fresh leaves of basil to a 250ml/ 8fl oz/1 cup boiling water and allow to steep for 10 minutes. Strain while still warm.

Headaches

The majority of headaches are caused by nasal congestion or sinusitis, eyestrain, fatigue or tension. They can also be caused by stress or worries, with muscle spasms in the neck and upper back leading to head pains.

WOOD BETONY AND LAVENDER TEA
These herbs soothe the nerves and are helpful for tension headaches. You could try chamomile, or lime blossom tea to relieve a headache.

INGREDIENTS

2.5ml/½ tsp dried wood betony
2.5ml/½ tsp dried lavender
200ml/7fl oz/scant cup boiling
   water

1 Put the herbs into a cup and leave to steep in the boiling water for up to ten minutes.

2 Strain and drink twice a day.

Caution: Do not take more than 5ml/1 tsp betony per day.

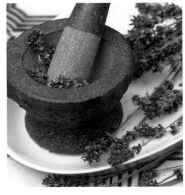

▲ LAVENDER HAS A DELICIOUS, UPLIFTING SCENT. USE IT TO PERFUME A BATH.

▼ RUB LAVENDER OR ROSEMARY OIL INTO YOUR TEMPLES TO RELIEVE A HEADACHE.

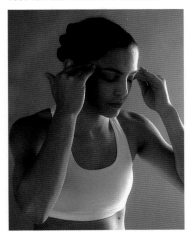

Herbal headache remedies

HANG A MUSLIN (CHEESECLOTH) BAG OF FRESH OR DRIED HERBS UNDER THE TAP WHEN YOU RUN A BATH.
MAKE A LAVENDER COMPRESS BY SOAKING SOFT COTTON FABRIC IN A LAVENDER INFUSION AND WRINGING IT OUT SLIGHTLY.

Hangovers

Most hangover symptoms – headache, nausea, fuzzy head and depression – are connected with the liver being unable to perform many of its functions. Bitter herbs can stimulate the liver, but avoid vervain if you suffer from liver disease.

MORNING-AFTER TEA

Vervain is bitter and lavender aids digestion; both lift the spirits.

INGREDIENTS

  5ml/1 tsp dried vervain
  2.5ml/½ tsp lavender flowers
  600ml/1 pint/2½ cups water

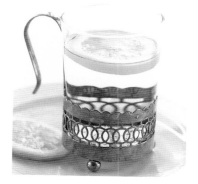

1 Bring the water to the boil and add the herbs. Cover the pan of boiling water to retain the volatile oils, and remove from the heat.

▲ IF YOU HAVE A HANGOVER, DRINK PLENTY OF WATER TO FLUSH THROUGH YOUR BODY, AND TAKE EXTRA VITAMIN C. A CUP OF BOILING WATER WITH A SLICE OF LEMON IN IT, OR FRESHLY SQUEEZED LEMON JUICE, WILL GIVE THE LIVER A BOOST.

2 Allow to steep for ten minutes. Strain and sweeten with a little honey. Sip a cup of this tea slowly.

▼ HERBAL TEAS ARE EXCELLENT CLEANSERS.

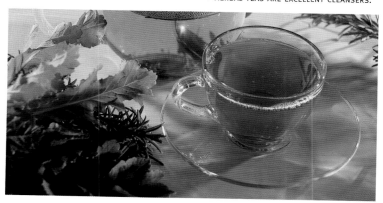

Migraines

These are more than a severe headache. They generally involve acute pains, often over one eye, and perhaps distorted vision or flashing lights. There may also cause nausea or vomiting and sensitivity to bright lights.

NECK MASSAGE FOR MIGRAINE
Use rosemary essential oil to massage your neck with. Keep your arms relaxed while massaging.

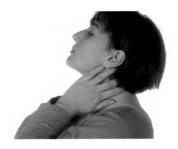

1 For stiff, aching neck muscles massage the neck with firm circular movements.

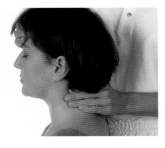

2 Ideally have someone else massage your neck for you. They can support your head while massaging.

Herbal tea remedies to relieve migraines

CHOOSE FROM CHAMOMILE OR ROSEMARY, ACCORDING TO YOUR TYPE OF MIGRAINE. MAKE AN INFUSION OR TEA WITH THE CHOSEN HERB AND SIP IT THROUGHOUT THE DAY.

CHAMOMILE IS GOOD FOR A DULL, THROBBING HEADACHE WITH A FEELING OF QUEASINESS – ADD A LITTLE GINGER TO RELIEVE MORE SEVERE NAUSEA.

FEVERFEW RELIEVES THE FEELING OF A TIGHT BAND AROUND THE HEAD. IT IS ALSO AVAILABLE IN TABLET FORM.

ROSEMARY HELPS WHERE STRESS IS A TRIGGER FOR MIGRAINES AND WHERE LOCAL WARMTH GIVES RELIEF.

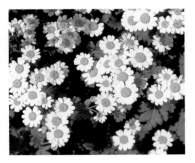

▲ FEVERFEW LEAVES ARE VERY BITTER. THE BEST WAY TO TAKE THEM IS SANDWICHED BETWEEN TWO SLICES OF BREAD.

Tense muscles

When we are anxious, we raise our shoulders and contract our back muscles. The effort of maintaining our muscles in this way is tiring. Tight neck muscles can also partially restrict blood flow to the head and so bring on a headache.

COLD-INFUSED LAVENDER OIL
This recipe is easy to make and very versatile. You could make marjoram or rosemary oils in the same way.

INGREDIENTS
> dried lavender heads
> clear vegetable oil

1 Fill a jar with lavender heads and cover completely with oil. Replace the lid. Allow to steep in a sunny place for a month. Shake daily.

2 Strain and bottle. Massage into stiff muscles or add to your bath to encourage relaxation.

CAUTION
• Do not use concentrated essential oil on your skin, dilute it by adding 2 drops of oil to 20ml/4 tsp of grapeseed or almond oil.

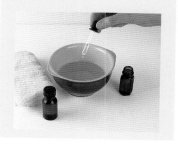

▼ IF YOU SPEND A LOT OF TIME STANDING OR SITTING IN THE SAME POSITION YOU NEED TO KEEP STRETCHING AND RELAXING YOUR LIMBS.

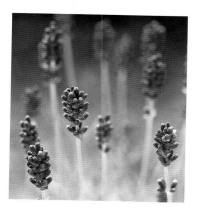

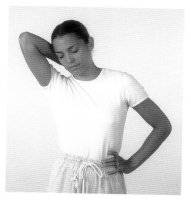

Insomnia

It is important to distinguish between habitual sleeplessness and temporary insomnia caused by worry. Do not become obsessed with trying to get a certain amount of sleep; not everyone needs eight hours.

LAVENDER TINCTURE

Store tinctures in dark bottles in a cool place for best results.

INGREDIENTS

15g/½oz dried lavender
250ml/8fl oz/1 cup vodka, made up to 300ml/½ pint/1¼ cups with water

1 Put the lavender into a glass jar and pour in the vodka and water. Put a lid on the jar and leave in a cool, dark place for ten days (no longer), shaking occasionally. The tincture turns dark purple.

2 Strain off the lavender through a muslin before pouring into a sterilized glass bottle. Seal with a cork.

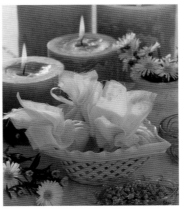

▲ TRY FILLING A MUSLIN (CHEESECLOTH) BAG WITH LAVENDER AND HOLD IT UNDER THE WATER FLOWING FROM THE BATH TAP. ADD LIGHTED CANDLES TO HELP CREATE MOOD.

▼ TAKE TIME TO UNWIND BEFORE YOU GO TO BED. LISTEN TO SOOTHING MUSIC AND TREAT THE EYES TO A CUCUMBER FACIAL.

Herbal insomnia remedies

MAKE THE HERBS LISTED BELOW INTO TINCTURES OR USE THE DRIED HERB TUCKED UNDER YOUR PILLOW.

CHAMOMILE	LAVENDER
HYSSOP	LEMON BALM
LIME BLOSSOM	VIOLET
PASSIONFLOWER	

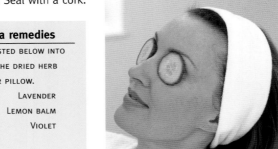

Stress

Stress in itself is not harmful and can in fact be motivating. But when the amount of stress is too much for our system to cope with, then it can cause other more harmful medical conditions.

STRESS-BUSTER TEA

Choose relaxing infusions from herbs such as lavender, lime blossom, lemon balm and valerian. A mixture of vervain, rosemary and betony (no more than 2.5ml/½ tsp per cup) are a tonic for exhaustion.

INGREDIENTS

*30ml/2 tbsp fresh or 15ml/
1 tbsp dried herb
600ml/1 pint/2½ cups boiling
water*

1 Put the herbs and water in a teapot. Steep for ten minutes.

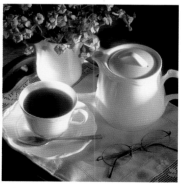

▲ AVOID CAFFEINE WHEN YOU ARE STRESSED. CHOOSE HEALTHY HERBAL TEAS INSTEAD.

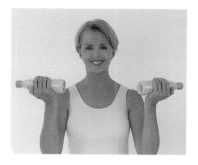

▲ EXERCISE HELPS TO REMOVE TENSION AND CHANGES THE FOCUS OF YOUR ATTENTION.

SYMPTOMS OF STRESS
• Constantly on edge and on the verge of tears.
• Difficulty in concentrating.
• Always tired, even after a night's sleep, and unable to relax or unwind – even if not working.
• Feelings of being unable to cope with life.
• Poor appetite or else nibbling without hunger.
• No sense of fun or enjoyment.
• Mistrustful of everybody.
• Problems in relationships, no interest in sex.
• Always fidgeting or biting nails or chewing hair.

Acidity and heartburn

Bouts of acidity and heartburn may occur after consuming rich foods or eating too quickly, and can be a symptom of indigestion. If the condition is temporary, make teas from the suggested herbs. Seek help if the problem persists.

MEADOWSWEET TINCTURE
This herb is a traditional remedy for heartburn, gastric ulcers and excess acidity.
INGREDIENTS
115g/4oz dried, or 300g/11oz freshly picked meadowsweet flowers
250ml/8fl oz/1 cup vodka
250ml/8fl oz/1 cup water

1 Place the herb flowers in a jar. Pour in the vodka and water.

2 Put a tight-fitting lid on the jar and leave to steep for a month, preferably on a sunny windowsill. Gently shake the jar.

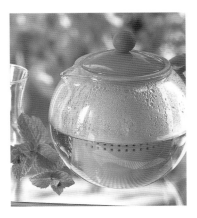

▲ PEPPERMINT TEA IS A GOOD TEA TO TAKE FOR INDIGESTION AND ACIDITY.

3 Strain and store the tincture in a dark glass bottle (it will keep for up to 18 months).

4 Take 5ml/1 tsp, three times a day, diluted in a little water or fruit juice.

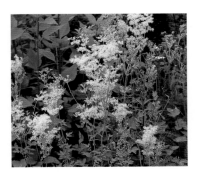

◀ GROW MEADOWSWEET IN YOUR GARDEN AND ADD THE LEAVES TO STEWS OR SOUPS IF YOU ARE PRONE TO HEARTBURN.

Herbal teas for acidity and heartburn

CHAMOMILE	LEMON BALM
MEADOWSWEET	SLIPPERY ELM

Abscesses

An abscess is a localized, inflamed swelling containing pus which can develop externally on the skin or internally in the mouth or other mucous membranes – the latter should be treated by a medical professional.

HOT MARSHMALLOW POULTICE

A poultice made of marshmallow to heal an inflammation is one of the earliest recorded uses for a herb.

INGREDIENTS

> *2 handfuls fresh marshmallow leaves or 15ml/1 tbsp powdered marshmallow root*
> *250ml/8fl oz/1 cup of boiling water or about 45ml/3 tbsp of hot water*
> *olive or almond oil*

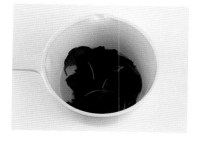

1 Pour the boiling water over the leaves in a bowl. If you are using powdered root, mix it with a little hot water to make a paste.

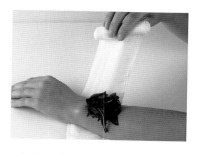

2 Apply a little oil to the skin in the affected area first, so that the poultice does not stick and burn the skin. Place the leaves or the paste on the abscess and cover with clean gauze or strips of cotton, lint or muslin.

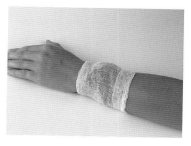

3 Hold in position with tape or a safety pin. You can keep the poultice on for several hours but may need to replace the contents of it every couple of hours. It may feel a little damp and uncomfortable to begin with.

Bites and stings

Summary brings a host of insects such as bees, wasps and hornets that can sting. In any situation where a bite or sting affects the mouth or throat, or if there are signs of an allergic reaction, get medical help immediately.

MARIGOLD INFUSION

Only the pot marigold *Calendula officinalis* has a medicinal value, so make sure you choose the right one when picking your flowers.

INGREDIENTS

heatproof bowl

1 litre/1¾ pints/4 cups boiling water

20 marigold flower-heads

1 Warm the bowl. Place the flowers in the bowl and pour over the just-boiled water. Cover with a tea towel and leave to stand for ten minutes.

2 Strain the liquid into a bottle. Apply the infusion as a skin lotion or on a cold compress to ease the pain of a bite or sting.

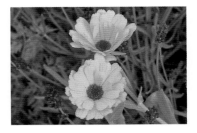

REMOVING A STING

Some stings, for instance those of bees, result in the sting being left behind in the skin. This should be carefully removed before applying any ointments or herbal treatments to the affected area. Try using a pair of tweezers if you cannot steady your hand. But take care, not to burst the poison sac when removing the sting, as this will send more toxin into the puncture, causing further irritation.

Bite and sting remedies

COMPRESS – WORMWOOD, WITCH HAZEL, CHAMOMILE, ELDERFLOWER, RED CLOVER, MARIGOLD, LAVENDER, LEMON BALM, PLANTAIN, YELLOW DOCK.

FRESH HERBS – ALOE VERA, HOUSELEEK, LEMON BALM, BASIL, DOCK LEAF, ONION.

OINTMENT – CHICKWEED, MARIGOLD.

POULTICE – CARROT (FOR SUNBURN), OATMEAL.

TINCTURE – ST JOHN'S WORT.

◀ MARIGOLD IS USED IN SKIN CREAMS TO SOOTHE AND HEAL.

Cuts, grazes and bruises

Before treating any cuts, grazes and bruises, make sure that the affected area is properly cleaned with water and a clean cloth to remove any dirt. An ointment will help to draw out dirt that is deeply embedded in the skin.

COMFREY BRUISE OINTMENT
Apply this ointment to varicose veins, bruises and inflamed muscles.
INGREDIENTS
> *200g/7oz petroleum jelly or paraffin wax*
> *25g/1oz fresh comfrey leaves*

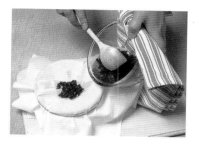

1 Put the petroleum jelly in a bowl. Set it over a pan of boiling water, add the chopped comfrey leaves and stir well. Heat over gently simmering water for about one hour.

2 Strain the mixture through muslin secured to the rim of a bowl with a rubber band. Gradually pour the liquid into a clean glass jar, before it has chance to set.

Herbal remedies for cuts and grazes

COMPRESS – WITCH HAZEL (THOUGH NOT ON BROKEN SKIN).
OINTMENT – MARIGOLD, COMFREY.
POULTICE – SAGE.
TINCTURE – MARIGOLD, MYRRH, YARROW.

Herbal remedies for bruises

COMPRESS – WITCH HAZEL, COMFREY, WORMWOOD.
ESSENTIAL OILS – LAVENDER.
OINTMENT – HOUSELEEK, YARROW.
POULTICE – COMFREY.

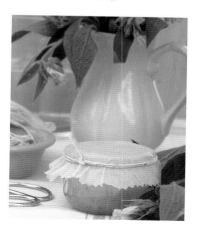

▲ USE COMFREY SPARINGLY AND NEVER TAKE IT INTERNALLY.

Burns and sunburn

Severe burns require medical assistance. The immediate treatment is to apply cold water for up to ten minutes to reduce the heat. With sunburn, be sure to avoid further exposure to the sun until all the symptoms have cleared.

AFTER SUN SOOTHING OIL

A cooling oil for burnt skin.

INGREDIENTS

   5 drops rose essential oil
   5 drops chamomile essential oil
   45ml/3 tbsp grapeseed oil
   45ml/3 tbsp virgin olive oil
   15ml/1 tbsp wheatgerm oil

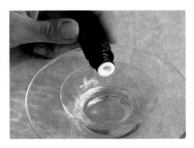

1 Combine the oils in a small bowl. Massage gently into the burn.

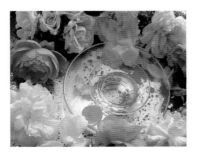

MARIGOLD OINTMENT FOR BURNS

This ointment moisturizes and soothes the skin.

INGREDIENTS

   200g/7oz petroleum jelly
   about 25g/1oz marigold flower
    heads, roughly chopped

1 Put the petroleum jelly in a bowl. Set it over a pan of boiling water, add the marigolds and stir. Heat over simmering water for one hour.

2 Strain the mixture through muslin secured to the rim of a jug with a rubber band. Pour the liquid immediately into a clean glass jar, before it has a chance to set. Leave to cool then refrigerate.

TIPS

• Aloe vera gel is an excellent first-aid treatment for burns. Break open a leaf and spread the gel directly on to the burn.
• You could also try infusions of elderflower, rose, chamomile, lavender, and tea tree.

Halitosis and mouth ulcers

Bad breath can result from several things such as an upset stomach, or teeth that need cleaning. For an instant breath freshener chew fresh parsley after a meal. Mouth ulcers are an indication of being run down. Herbs can help both.

SAGE AND SALT TOOTHPOWDER

This toothpaste replacement will clean your teeth and keep your breath fresh.

INGREDIENTS

    25g/1oz sage leaves
    60ml/4 tbsp sea salt

1 Shred the sage leaves into an ovenproof dish using scissors.

2 Mix in the salt, grinding it into the leaves with a pestle. Bake in a very low oven for about one hour until crisp.

3 Pound the baked ingredients until reduced to powder. Use in place of toothpaste on a damp toothbrush.

Herbal mouth ulcer tinctures

MYRHH	MARIGOLD
RASPBERRY LEAF	SAGE
THYME	

Herbal teeth cleansers

RUB TEETH WITH FRESH SAGE LEAVES.

MYRRH AND SAGE MOUTH ULCER RINSE

Sage has antiseptic qualities and is a good herb for mouth complaints.

INGREDIENTS

    15ml/1tbsp dried sage
    100ml/½ pint/1¼ cups boiling water
    10ml/2 tsp tincture of myrrh

1 Put the sage leaves in a bowl. Pour the boiling water over. Leave to stand for 20 minutes, strain and mix in the myrrh. Allow to cool. Use to rinse your mouth.

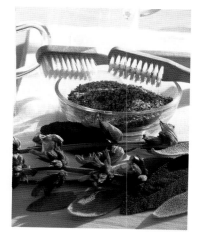

Acne and spots

Acne is caused by increasing levels of hormones, which, during the teens, cause the skin's glands to overproduce sebum (the natural oily skin lubricant), blocking the pores. Regular cleansing will help to remove this oily excess.

FEVERFEW COMPLEXION MILK

Feverfew is easy to grow in the garden and self-seeds prodigiously. When the leaves are heated with milk, they produce an excellent tonic which, once applied to the skin, helps to clear blemishes, discourage blackheads and moisturize dry skin.

INGREDIENTS
1 large handful of feverfew
leaves
600ml /1 pint /2½ cups milk
A saucepan, strainer and bottle

1 Place the feverfew leaves and milk into a small pan, bring to the boil, then reduce the heat and simmer for 20 minutes.

2 Remove the pan from the heat and allow the mixture to cool. Strain into a bottle and store in the refrigerator until needed.

3 Apply cold to the skin, taking care to massage in thoroughly.

▼ FEVERFEW LEAVES CAN BE USED BOTH TO CLEANSE AND MOISTURIZE FACIAL SKIN.

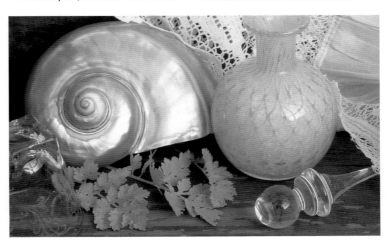

Dry and sore lips

It is quite simple to make your own soothing cream for lips chapped by sun, wind, weather or illness. You can also apply a simple mixture of honey and rosewater as a salve for sore or chapped lips.

LAVENDER LIP BALM

Beeswax and cocoa butter are rich emollients; lavender oil is well known for its healing ability.

INGREDIENTS

> *5ml/1 tsp beeswax*
> *5ml/1 tsp cocoa butter*
> *5ml/1 tsp wheatgerm oil*
> *5ml/1 tsp almond oil*
> *3 drops lavender essential oil*

1 Put all but the last ingredient, into a bowl and set over a pan of simmering water. Stir until melted.

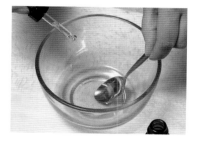

2 Remove from the heat and allow to cool for a few minutes before mixing in the lavender oil. Pour into a small jar and leave to set.

▼ BEESWAX HAS A HIGH MELTING POINT, SO BE PATIENT.

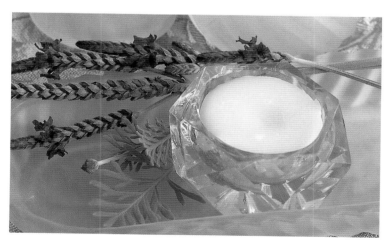

Dry and oily skin

Moisturizing cream prevents dryness of the skin, keeps wrinkles at bay and protects your skin from the weather. If you like, substitute pot marigolds for the elderflowers. Splash a little tonic on to your face first to feel refreshed.

DRY SKIN MOISTURIZER
Elderflowers have a reputation for lightening dry skin. Store this face cream in the refrigerator. It keeps for several months.

INGREDIENTS
    120ml/4fl oz/½ cup water
    10ml/2 tsps dried elderflowers
    30ml/2 tbsp emulsifying
      ointment
    5ml/1 tsp beeswax
    30ml/2 tbsp almond oil
    2.5ml/½ tsp borax

1 Boil the water and pour over the dried elderflowers in a jar. Leave to stand for 30 minutes then strain.

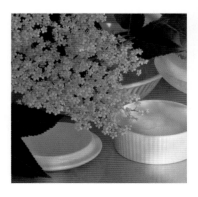

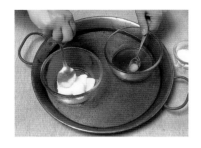

2 Put the emulsifying ointment, beeswax and almond oil into one bowl and the elderflower infusion and borax into another. Set both over hot water and stir until the oils melt and the borax dissolves.

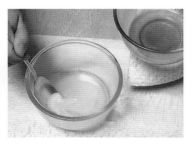

3 Remove from the heat and pour the elderflower mixture into the oils. Stir gently until incorporated. Leave to cool, stirring at intervals. Pour into a jar before it sets.

ELDERFLOWER SKIN TONIC

This refreshing skin tonic can be made to suit your skin type and should be applied to your face direct from the refrigerator. It keeps for a few days, or can be frozen in small quantities and thawed as required.

INGREDIENTS

10 dried elderflower heads
300ml/½ pint/1¼ cups still bottled water, boiled
15ml/1 tbsp either cider vinegar for normal skin, or witch hazel for slightly oily skin, or vodka for very oily skin

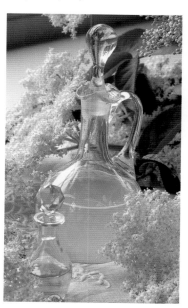

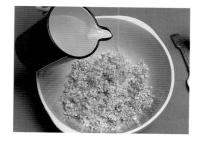

1 Strip the elderflowers from the stems and place in a bowl. Pour the boiling water over the flowers. Cover with a tea towel and leave for 20 minutes. Add either the cider vinegar, witch hazel or vodka, cover and leave overnight to infuse.

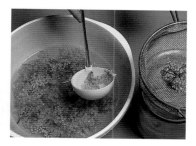

2 Strain into a sterilized jar, cover and allow to cool. Store chilled.

Mint and marigold moisturizer for oily skin

USE 25G/1OZ FRESH MINT LEAVES WITH 15G/½OZ FRESH MARIGOLD PETALS AND 600ML/1 PINT/2½ CUPS BOILING WATER WITH 30ML/2 TBSP VODKA.

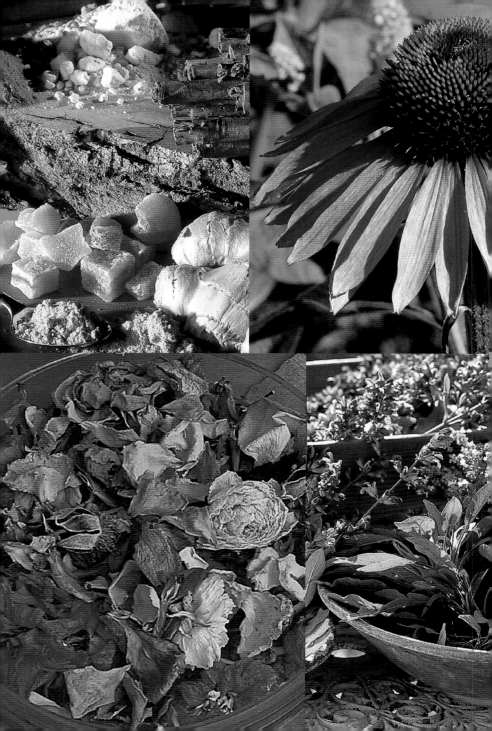

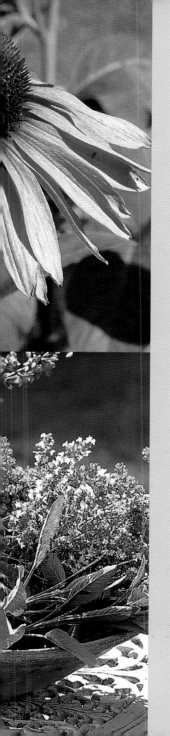

HEALING PLANTS
DIRECTORY

This directory features up to 80 of the best-known healing flowers and herbs, many of which can be grown easily at home. There is information on characteristics such as height and leaf shape, to help you to identify them, plus advice on how to use the various parts of each plant to heal safely and effectively.

Special care should be taken when using flowers or herbs as part of internal remedies. It is essential that you use the correct dosage as prescribed by a qualified herbalist, and, if pregnant or taking other medicines, discuss usage with a medical professional. Remember that plant remedies do not work instantly, so give them time to take effect. Seek further medical advice if symptoms persist.

The directory

Achillea millefolium,
YARROW
Pungent perennial herb with flat, whitish or pink flowerheads and feathery leaves. The essential oil can treat catarrh; the bitter-tasting infusion sweats out colds and fevers. Yarrow is also used externally to treat wounds, nose-bleeds and as a skin toner.

Agrimonia eupatoria,
AGRIMONY
Perennial herb with yellow flower spikes which, when dried, can be used in anti-inflammatory, anti-bacterial infusions. Used internally to treat sore throats, catarrh, diarrhoea, cystitis and urinary infections. Forms the basis of lotions used to treat skin wounds and stem external bleeding.

Allium sativum,
GARLIC
This versatile herb has many medicinal properties and can be taken orally in a variety of forms. It helps to lower blood pressure and reduce blood cholesterol, and is thought to inhibit blood clotting which leads to circulatory diseases. Garlic is also used as a decongestant, and has strong antiseptic properties.

Aloe vera,
ALOE VERA
The fleshy, spiny-toothed leaves of this famous plant ooze a thick gel which is used in a whole host of health and beauty treatments. Aloe vera contains various anti-inflammatory agents, minerals, anti-oxidant vitamins C, E, B12 and beta carotene. The gel from the leaves is applied to burns, bites, bruises and skin irritations.

Althaea officinalis,
MARSHMALLOW
Hardy perennial with pale pink flowers. Flowers and roots are famed for soothing, sweet mucilage, and as lozenges relieve inflamed gums, mouth and gastric ulcers, and bronchial infections. Used externally, the flowers help to soothe inflamed skin. The modern confectionery of the same name no longer contains the herb.

Anemone pulsatilla,
PASQUE FLOWER

A hardy perennial with bell-shaped purplish-blue flowers, followed by silky seedheads. Pasque is used for treating menstrual cramps, PMS, and in remedies for male reproductive problems. The flowers are usually prescribed in homeopathic rather than fresh form, as the plant can be toxic. **Caution:** Avoid usage during pregnancy.

Anethum graveolens,
DILL

An aromatic annual with a soft, feathery texture. Dill is a cooling, soothing herb which, taken orally, aids digestion and constipation, and is also used to treat inflammation. Poultices made from the leaves soothe boils and ease swellings and joint pains. The seeds are chewed to cure bad breath.

Arnica montana,
ARNICA

An alpine perennial with cheerful, yellow, daisy-like flowers. Used internally to relieve shock and pain, and to prevent colds, but should only be taken in prescribed, homeopathic doses as can be toxic in excess. Arnica is also used externally as part of a soothing lotion for bruises and sprains.

Artemisia absinthium,
WORMWOOD

Perennial shrub with hairy stems and aromatic, downy, grey-green leaves. To taste, wormwood is extremely bitter (*absinthium* means "without sweetness"). It is a strong tonic for the digestive system but can be toxic if used in excess. It is useful for curing anaemia, easing wind and during periods of recuperation.

Borago officinalis,
BORAGE

Hairy annual plant with bristly leaves and mauve, star-shaped flowers. As a herbal infusion it can be applied to inflamed skin, and flowers produce a safe, essential oil used to treat hormonal problems and PMS. The flowers can be taken as tea to dispel depression and nervous anxiety.

Calamintha nepeta,
CALAMINT
A bushy perennial mint with tubular, pink-mauve flowers. Leaves and flower tops are used as a stimulating tea or as a tonic or infusion for settling wind and indigestion. **Caution:** Avoid usage during pregnancy.

Calendula officinalis,
MARIGOLD
The marigold, or pot marigold, is a low-growing annual with cheerful orange-yellow petals. Herb is antiseptic, anti-inflammatory, anti-bacterial and anti-fungal. Added to soothing ointments for burns, eczema, sunburn, stings and bites. Has many benefits for the skin: use in an infusion to refresh tired skin, or add to hand and face cream to nourish and protect.

Carthamus tinctorius,
SAFFLOWER
Hardy annual with shaggy, thistle-like, red-yellow flowerheads and long ovate leaves. A tea, infused from fresh or dried flowers, induces perspiration, helping to reduce fevers, and is mildy laxative. Infusions can also be applied externally to treat bruises, skin irritations, inflammation and measles. **Caution:** Avoid usage during pregnancy.

Centaurea cyanus,
CORNFLOWER
Tall annual, with bright blue shaggy flowerheads. The flowers were used traditionally to make eyewashes for tired or strained eyes, but are more commonly prized today for their aromatic properties. The petals produce a bitter tonic, and the mildly laxative seeds help to relieve constipation in children.

Chamaemelum nobile,
CHAMOMILE
Evergreen perennial with feathery leaves and white daisy-like flowers. This antiseptic and anti-inflammatory plant is soothing when used as an infusion or essential oil. The famous tea alleviates nausea, indigestion and promotes sleep. As a steam inhalation, it eases asthma, sinusitis or catarrh.

Citrus aurantium,
BITTER ORANGE
This evergreen tree with shiny, ovate leaves produces a fragrant white blossom and bitter orange fruits. Essential oil can be made from all three components: neroli from the flowers, oil of petitgrain from the leaves and twigs, and oil of orange from the rind. Oils are rich in vitamins A, B and C, and have a calming effect. **Caution:** None of the essential oils given above should be taken internally.

Cnicus benedictus,
HOLY THISTLE
Annual with red, hairy stems, spiny leaves and yellow flowers. Leaves and tops are used for their antiseptic, antibiotic qualities, but are very bitter. Infusion or tincture is an effective tonic, and can help to stimulate the appetite. Holy thistle was traditionally used for fevers and settling stomach.

Crataegus laevigata,
HAWTHORN
Common deciduous shrub/small tree, with thorny branches. Produces white, scented flowers and red, globe-shaped fruits, known as haws. Bioflavonoid content makes it a valuable, slow-working "food for the heart". It lowers blood pressure and eases hypertension.

Crocus sativus,
SAFFRON CROCUS
A perennial crocus which produces lilac flowers with three red styles. The styles are dried to make saffron, which is known to have digestive properties, improve circulation and reduce high blood pressure. It is used widely in cooking and is a rich source of vitamin B2.

Echinacea purpurea
CONEFLOWER
Hardy perennial with large pinkish-purple, daisy-like flowers. The dried roots are made into capsules and powders to treat the common cold. Recent research has shown echinadea to have a beneficial effect on the immune system. Taken as a tea, it helps kidney infections, or is used as a compress for boils and abscesses.

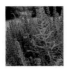 *Echium vulgare*,
VIPER'S BUGLOSS
A bushy and bristly biennial with prickly leaves and violet-blue flowers. In medieval times it was held that, because it resembled a snake's skin and tongue, it must be an antidote to adder bite or other poisons. Today, it is used for its skin-healing abilities. **Caution:** May cause stomach upset if ingested, and irritate the skin upon first contact. To be used by qualified herbalists only.

 Eschscholzia californica,
CALIFORNIA POPPY
Annual or perennial poppy with bright orange, yellow or pink flowers. A sedative plant that relieves pain and is taken internally as an infusion, for anxiety, nervous tension and insomnia. Good for children, for bedwetting or sleeping problems.

 Eupatorium cannabinum,
HEMP AGRIMONY
A hard and woody perennial with red stem and pinkish-white flowers (a local name was "raspberries and cream"). Used as a diuretic and as a tonic and for flu-like illnesses. Its alkaloid content means that caution should be exercised in usage. Applied externally to ulcers and sores.

 Euphrasia officinalis,
EYEBRIGHT
An annual, semi-parasitic herb which grows on grasses and has white flowers double-lipped with yellow throats. Infusion used externally as a bath for sore or itchy eyes, skin irritations; internally it helps to relieve hayfever, allergic rhinitis, catarrh and sinusitis.

 Filipendula ulmaria,
MEADOWSWEET
This perennial of damp meadows has sweet-smelling creamy flowers and was traditionally used to make aspirin. Both leaves and flowers are now used as an infusion for excess acid, gastric ulcers, rheumatism, arthritis and urinary infections. Safe remedy for children with upset stomachs.

Galega officinalis,
GOAT'S RUE
A bushy perennial with mauve, white or bicoloured flowers resembling those of a sweetpea. Has sedative properties, and infusions are taken to relieve irritability and insomnia. A diuretic, it can improve liver function and has a tonic effect on the system.

Galium odoratum or *Asperula odorata,*
SWEET WOODRUFF
Spreading perennial with spear-shaped leaves and small, white star-shaped flowers. Used as infusion for soothing nerves and insomnia, as a diuretic to improve liver function, and for varicose veins. **Caution:** Avoid usage during pregnancy.

Geranium maculatum,
CRANESBILL
Hardy perennial with round, purplish-pink flowers, native to North America. Whole plant dried for infusions, powders and tinctures; used as astringent to control bleeding and discharges, for diarrhoea and haemorrhoids. Used externally for wounds and as gargle for sore throats and mouth ulcers.

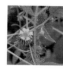

Geum urbanum,
WOOD AVENS
A hardy perennial with small, five-petalled yellow flowers. Whole plant is used: the flowers in infusions, the roots in decoctions. Treats digestive upsets, sore gums and mouth inflammations; can also be used externally to remedy haemorrhoids. The old name, herb bennet, recalls "benedict" (blessed) and the belief that it repelled evil spirits.

Glycyrrhiza glabra,
LICORICE
A plant with ovate leaves and long seed pods, licorice is famed for its use in confectionery. The root has more active medicinal properties, and as an anti-inflammatory agent is used to soothe stomach disorders, sore throats and respiratory infections. **Caution:** Seek advice before using as can raise blood pressure. Avoid usage during pregnancy.

Helianthus annuus,
SUNFLOWER
Tall, impressive and showy annual with large yellow flowerheads and brown disc florets at the centre. The whole plant is used for extracts and tinctures; the seeds are used in the production of sunflower oil. This is an excellent source of vitamin E (an anti-oxidant) and polyunsaturates, which maintain cell membranes and lower blood cholesterol.

Hypericum perforatum,
ST JOHN'S WORT
The yellow flowering tops of this plant are used fresh or dried in infusions, creams and oils. Has antiseptic and anti-inflammatory properties and can be applied to ease burns and muscular pain, including sciatica. Although originally prescribed as an anti-depressant, research now suggests that St John's wort may interact adversely with many other prescribed medicines. **Caution:** Should never be taken internally without first consulting a qualified medical practitioner.

Hyssopus officinalis,
HYSSOP
Semi-evergreen with flowers in blue-pink spikes. Leaves and flowers used in infusions, as an expectorant, for promoting sweating and as an anti-catarrhal and anti-bacterial remedy. Its essential oil is restricted in some countries.

Jasminum officinale,
JASMINE
Evergreen rambler, with sweet-scented white flowers used in calming infusions. The essential oil is used externally on dry skin and in the bath or massage oil. **Caution:** Oil should not be taken internally.

Lavandula angustifolia,
LAVENDER
Cultivated for so long that it now has numerous hybrids, common lavender was the first aromatherapy oil and remains an excellent first aid remedy for skin problems, headaches and nervous digestion. Taken in tea, it relieves headaches and promotes sleep.

Leonurus cardiaca,
MOTHERWORT
A pungent perennial with mauve-pink, double-lipped flowering tops, used in infusions and tinctures. Mildly sedative, with a calming effect on the heart and on palpitations. **Caution:** Avoid usage during pregnancy.

Lilium candidum,
MADONNA LILY
This perennial has pure white, fragrant, trumpet-shaped flowers. The juice from the roots and flowers is used externally in ointments to treat burns, and skin inflammations and disorders.

Lonicera periclymenum,
HONEYSUCKLE
Hardy climber with fragrant, creamy white or yellow flowers, followed by poisonous red berries in Autumn. The leaves were traditionally favoured as an expectorant, the bark as a diuretic and the flowers for asthma. These days its chief use is as a Bach remedy for nostalgia.

Lycopus europaeus,
GIPSYWEED
A perennial mint-like herb which lacks aroma. Astringent and sedative, gipsyweed was once used to treat haemorrhaging, palpitations and menstrual problems; still thought to have sedative properties. Its black dye, said to be used by gypsies to darken their skin, gave this plant its common name.

Lythrum salicaria,
PURPLE LOOSESTRIFE
A perennial with erect stems and crimson-purple flowers. Continues to be recommended by modern herbalists for relief of diarrhoea, dysentery, haemorrhaging and excessive menstrual flow.

Marrubium vulgare,
HOREHOUND
Hardy, tall perennial with small white flowers, and a common weed. Usage is controlled by law in some countries. The stems are used as a bitter infusion for non-productive coughs, colds and chest infections.

Melaleuca alternifolia,
Tea-tree
Evergreen with thin, pointed and leathery leaves, and bottle-brush shaped flowers. An antiseptic, anti-bacterial and antifungal, the oil is diluted in carrier oil and used externally to treat burns, stings, insect bites and acne. Undiluted, it is said to be effective against dermatological conditions such as warts and verrcuas.

Melilotus officinalis,
Melilot
An erect, straggly biennial with yellow, honey-scented flowers. Dried flowering stems are used in infusions or tinctures, as a sedative and anti-inflammatory agent, to treat sleeplessness, tension headaches, flatulence and menopause. **Caution:** If improperly dried, the plant is toxic. Consult a qualified practitioner before use.

Melissa officinalis,
Lemon balm
The rough-textured green leaves of this busy perennial release a fresh lemony scent when crushed. Infusions of the fresh leaves are sedative and soothing, good for treating headaches, indigestion, nervous tension, anxiety and depression. Externally, it can be used in creams to soothe the skin or as an insect repellent.

Mentha,
Mint
There are many varieties of mint and each has its own properties. Peppermint is taken as a tea for colds, and to aid digestion. The essential oil has decongestant properties and can be used as an inhalant to relieve colds, chest infections, catarrh and asthma.

Monarda didyma,
Bergamot
An aromatic hardy perennial with red or mauve flowers. A native of North America, the leaves were made into Oswego tea by early settlers. Bergamot essential oil, extracted from the bergamot orange, *Citrus bergamia*, is still used to flavour Earl Grey tea. The leaves and flowers aid digestion.

Nepeta cataria,
CATMINT

A hardy perennial mint with coarse leaves and whitish-mauve flowers, irresistible to cats. An anti-inflammatory and mild sedative, leaves, flowers and stems make an infusion for feverish colds; used externally for cuts and bruises. Mild enough for children.

Ocimum basilicum,
BASIL

This aromatic annual has soft, ovate, bright-green leaves. Basil has soothing, antiseptic properties and leaves are best used fresh. They can be rubbed on to insect bites, used in steam inhalations, or made into cough syrups with a little honey. Basil produces a safe essential oil which is used in massage, and to treat anxiety.

Oenothera biennis,
EVENING PRIMROSE

Not related to the primrose, this plant is so named because its bright yellow flowers open in the evening. The seeds are pressed to produce an oil which is used for boosting the immune system and hormones. It is taken internally for PMS, menopause and allergies, and externally for skin tone.

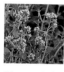

Origanum majorana,
SWEET MARJORAM

Half-hardy aromatic perennial with small lilac pink clusters of flowers. A warming, relaxing, antiseptic herb, it is taken internally as an infusion to treat nervous tension, headaches, insomnia, bronchial complaints, digestive problems and painful periods. The essential oil is diluted and applied to stiff muscles, and joints.

Passiflora incarnata,
PASSION FLOWER

A hardy, tropical perennial climber, with a woody stem and creamy-white, or lavender-blue, intricate flowers. The whole plant is used in herbal medicine. Leaves and flowers are dried for use in infusions, tinctures and tablets. A gentle sedative, it is useful as a mild tranquillizer to treat nervous conditions and insomnia.

Pelargonium graveolens,
GERANIUM

A bushy aromatic perennial with pink flowers, also known as a rose geranium, this African flower is now a universal house plant. Contains a volatile oil used in perfumery, and dried leaves go into various scents and aromatics. Astringent and anti-depressant, it is good in teas for tension and exhaustion.

Petroselinum crispum,
PARSLEY

This well-known frost-hardy perennial grows on a short taproot and produces three-pinnate leaves. Parsley is rich in Vitamins A and E, and acts as an antioxidant. Parsley tea is sometimes used to treat coughs and jaundice, but it should not be used in excess as can be toxic.

Primula veris,
COWSLIP

A spring perennial bearing clusters of tubular yellow flowers. Becoming rare in the wild, but flowers and roots are used traditionally as part of a sedative infusion for children and as expectorant. Cowslip aids insomnia, chronic respiratory tract infections and also rheumatism. **Caution:** Avoid usage during pregnancy, or if taking aspirin.

Primula vulgaris,
PRIMROSE

A perennial with clusters of saucer-shaped, pale yellow flowers in early spring, primrose has similar healing properties to cowslip. Flowers (cultivated only, as wild form is rare and protected) are used as an infusion for easing anxiety, insomnia and respiratory tract problems.

Prunella vulgaris,
SELFHEAL

This aromatic herb has tall, violet, two-lipped florets which are dried for use in infusions, tinctures and ointments. Selfheal's common name reflects its traditional usage as a wound herb, to stop bleeding, for bites, bruises, sore throats and inflamed gums. It is still used to soothe burns, skin inflammations and sore gums.

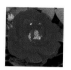

Rosa, ROSE
A deciduous bush of multiple types, roses have been used medicinally since antiquity as water, ointment, syrup, vinegar, conserve and candies. Their main therapeutic use is now in aromatherapy: the essential oil ("attar of roses") is used to relieve nervous depression and anxiety. Mildly sedative, rose essences are also used to treat sensitive skin and sore eyes. Rosehips, a rich source of Vitamin C, are used in cooking to make vinegars, syrups, wine and preserves. They can also be added to teas as a useful immunity booster.

Rosmarinus officinalis, ROSEMARY
This evergreen shrub, with aromatic, needle-like leaves and small pale blue flowers, is prized for its culinary, medicinal, aromatic and cosmetic uses. The leaves and flowers form the basis of infusions for colds, flu and headaches; tinctures for depression and nervous tension; essential oil for massages to relieve rheumatic, muscular pain;

in therapeutic baths to ease fatigue; and in hair products to reduce dandruff. **Caution:** Avoid usage during pregnancy.

Salvia, SAGE
An evergreen, highly aromatic shrub, sage has downy, rough-textured leaves which are both antiseptic and anti-bacterial. Use in a gargle or mouthwash for bad breath, or to treat sore throats, gums and mouth ulcers, and ease laryngitis and tonsillitis. Sage tea is a tonic that aids indigestion and menopausal problems. Applied externally as a compress, sage can help to treat wounds.

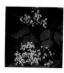

Sambucus nigra, ELDER
This small, deciduous tree produces creamy white flowers and clusters of black fruits. Infusions of the flowers are taken for colds, sinusitis, and hayfever; berries make cough syrups. The flowers can be used for home-made skin toners, and the leaves are used in insecticides. **Caution:** Leaves are toxic and should not be taken interally.

Solidago virgaurea,
GOLDEN ROD
This hardy perennial with branched stems and profuse spikes of yellow flowers has antioxidant, diuretic and astringent properties. The leaves and flowers are used to make lotions, ointments and poultices to treat wounds, bites and rashes. Internally, infusions help to ease urinary problems.

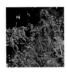

Stachys officinalis,
BETONY
A hardy perennial, with magenta-pink flowers. Both leaves and flowers were used historically in infusions, ointments and lotions to ease headaches. Its application today extends to remedies for anxiety and PMS. Externally, betony is good for cuts and bruises. **Caution:** Avoid usage in pregnancy and note that leaves are toxic if used in excess.

Symphytum officinale,
COMFREY
This wild, furry-leaved plant has blue or white flowers, and was historically used as a healing agent for fractures. Today, comfrey leaves are still used externally, as poultices, compresses and ointments to be applied to bruises, varicose veins, inflamed muscles and tendons.

Syzgium aromaticum,
CLOVE
A tropical evergreen which is named after the French word "clou", meaning nail, which the green buds (cloves) resemble. A stimulant, antiseptic and digestive remedy, it relieves nausea and controls vomiting. Oil of cloves is a dental analgesic, and sucking a clove can help to alleviate toothache.

Tanacetum parthenium,
FEVERFEW
With its green foliage and daisy-like flowers, this busy perennial is particularly successful in treating migraine – two or three leaves should be taken orally, with honey or another sweetener as they are very bitter. It is also taken in tablet form to ease rheumatism. **Caution:** Prolonged consumption may cause mouth ulcers.

Taraxacum officinale,
DANDELION
Perennial flowers with well-recognized yellow rosettes followed by fluffy seed heads in Autumn. Although dandelions are often thought of as growing in the wild, they are also cultivated for use in moist, fertile soil and the leaves and flowers have many medicinal properties, both fresh and dried. An effective diuretic, dandelion is taken internally for urinary infections and helps to treat diseases of the gall bladder and liver. It is also beneficial for rheumatic complaints and gout, and – while in itself a rich source of vitamins A and C, and of metals such as magnesium and iron – is said to promote appetite.

Tilia cordata,
LIME
This hardy, deciduous tree has heartshaped leaves and fluffy pale yellow flowers. Newly opened flowers are harvested and dried for linden teas, which are soothing and sweat-inducing. Mix with honey and lemon to treat colds, catarrh, fevers, anxiety and palpitations. Lime is also used to help combat high blood pressure.

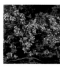

Thymus vulgaris,
THYME
There are many varieties of thyme, but *Thymus vulgaris*, with its white flowerheads, is the only one with acknowledged medicinal uses. As a mouthwash, it helps to combat mouth ulcers, and as a tea it soothes coughs, colds and sore throats. It also produces an essential oil that eases tense muscles, and a sachet of the dried leaves is used as an aid to sleep.

Trifolium pratense,
RED CLOVER
This rather short-lived perennial has pink, circular flowerheads which are used as part of an infusion of blossoms to treat coughs and eczema. Externally, the flowers are applied to skin complaints such as ulcers, burns and sores. Red clover was formerly used for cataracts as its white leaf halo suggested this "signature". Red clover is still used to help control blood sugar.

Tropaeolum majus,
NASTURTIUM
A half-hardy annual with circular leaves and yellow-orange single flowers. Native to Peru, it is widely used in Andean herbal medicine as a disinfectant and expectorant. The leaves, flowers and seeds are all edible, often used fresh to flavour salads and vinegars, and are high in vitamin C content. The seeds are anti-bacterial and can be used in infusions to clear urinary infections and catarrh.

Tussilago farfara,
COLTSFOOT
A small creeping perennial with cheering yellow blossoms which emerge in spring. The leaves or flowers of this herb contain a substance known as mucilage, which is used to produce soothing tonics for mucous membranes. Flavoursome and popular in salads, it is still used in infusions for coughs and can be applied externally, either as a paste of fresh leaves mixed with honey, or as a compress, to treat sores, ulcers and bites **Caution:** Avoid usage during pregnancy.

Urtica dioica,
STINGING NETTLE
A tough, spreading perennial covered in stinging hairs, the common nettle may be known as a bothersome weed, but for centuries it has been viewed as a nutritious and medicinal herb. Its high vitamin C content promotes the absorption of iron, which makes it a suitable remedy for anaemia. It is also diuretic, helping to rid the body of uric acid, promotes circulatory health, and can be used in a compress against rheumatoid aches. Decoctions of roots and leaves are applied to the scalp to alleviate dandruff, and it is even said to help prevent baldness.

Valeriana officinalis,
VALERIAN
Not to be confused with its other herbal relative, the purely ornamental red valerian (*Centranthus ruber*), this perennial with toothed leaflets and white, sometimes pinkish, flowers has strong sedative properties and can be taken as a tea for insomnia, headaches and nervous tension.

Verbena officinalis,
VERVAIN

A hardy, rather straggly perennial with dull green, slightly hairy leaves and small, sparse, lilac flowers, vervain was traditionally thought of as a holy herb (*herba sacra*), as it was supposedly used to staunch Christ's wounds at the Crucifixion. While still believed to have hypnotic and aphrodisiac powers, it is medicinally linked with disorders of the stomach, kidneys, liver, and gall bladder. Externally, vervain can be used in compresses and lotions for skin complaints, and as a gargle for sore gums and mouth ulcers.

Vinca major,
GREATER PERIWINKLE

A trailing evergreen perennial with glossy dark-green leaves and five-petalled violet blue flowers. Both the leaves and flowering stems are processed to extract an alkaloid which helps to dilate the blood vessels and reduce blood pressure. **Caution:** All parts of the plant are poisonous, and self-treatment is not advised.

Viola odorata,
SWEET VIOLET

A low-growing hardy perennial with a tall, basal rosette of heartshaped leaves and drooping flowers that yield an aromatherapy essential oil. Other parts of the plant make a gentle infusion or syrup for coughs, colds and rheumatism.

Viola tricolor,
WILD PANSY

Annual or perennial, with violet, yellow and white triangular flowers. Also known as heartsease, in reference to its older use as a heart tonic. Today, wild pansy is used in infusions as an expectorant for coughs and colds, and externally to treat skin complaints.

Zingiber officinale,
GINGER

Used in China since earliest times, this reed-like perennial has dense cones bearing yellow-green flowers. It is a stimulant, expectorant and antiseptic, often used as a cold remedy to promote sweating, eliminate toxins and dispel catarrh.

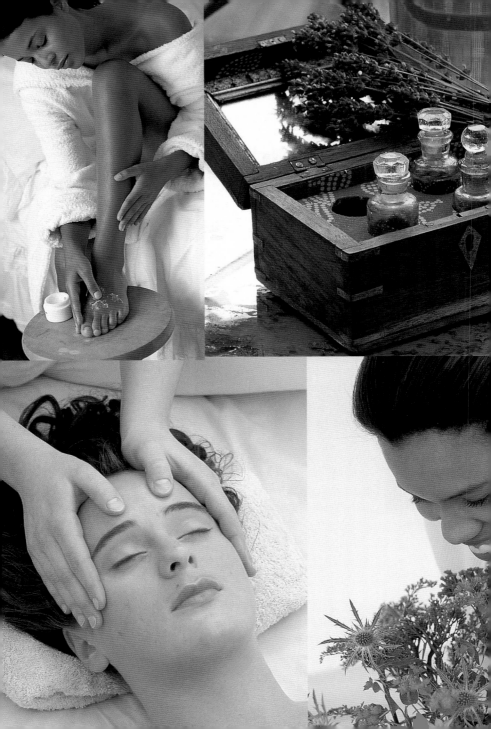

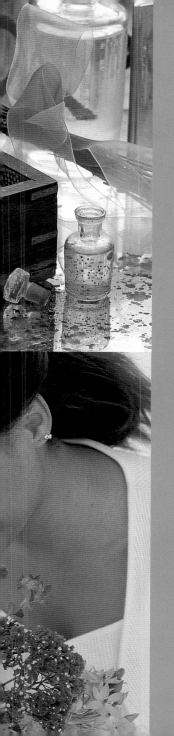

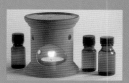

HEALING WITH
AROMA-
THERAPY

Since the dawn of human history, people have used scented products in religious ceremonies, bathing and massage, and for scenting the hair and body. In the 10th century, physicians learned how to distil essential oils from plants, and the practice of aromatherapy was born.

Essential oils can be extracted from a wide variety of plants, including citrus fruits, shrubs, vines, herbs and spices, and are used to relax, sedate, refresh or stimulate, according to need. In addition to affecting moods, however, these essential oils boast considerable healing powers and can soothe aches and ease skin conditions. It is not surprising, then, that so much use is made of aromatherapy in conventional medicine today.

Essential oils

Essential oils are natural, volatile substances that evaporate readily, releasing their aroma into the air, as happens, for example, when someone brushes against an aromatic plant. The oils have many beneficial properties.

A widely used method of employing essential oils in the home is to fragrance the rooms by means of a vaporizer or oil burner. Although vaporizers come in many forms, they all work on the same principle. The reservoir is filled with water, to which are added a few drops of essential oil. The reservoir is then heated, which causes the oil and water to evaporate. The heat must be fairly low to allow slow evaporation of the oil and a longer-lasting scent.

Adding a few drops of essential oil to a bowl of hot water is an effective way of adding scent to a room, especially in a dry atmosphere.

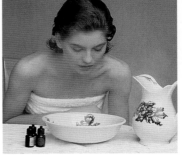

▲ ADD ESSENTIAL OILS TO HOT WATER FOR A BENEFICIAL STEAM INHALATION.

Choose an attractive bowl and place it out of reach of children. Use an oil that you really like, as its fragrance will linger for some time. You can also use the bowl of scented water for an uplifting or calming steam inhalation. Essential oils can be used to make a luxurious addition to the bath, whether they are chosen to aid recovery from an illness, to lift the spirits, or to promote relaxation after a stressful day.

▶ OIL BURNERS CAN MAKE ATTRACTIVE ROOM ORNAMENTS.

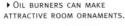

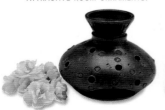

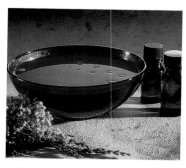

▲ A FEW DROPS OF ESSENTIAL OIL IN HOT WATER WILL PERFUME A ROOM.

The essential oils recommended for the bath affect the body as they are inhaled in the steam, but some also penetrate the skin pores that open in the warmth.

In order to add oils to the bath safely it is important to dilute them in vegetable oil, cream or full-fat (whole) milk. Add the blend to the bathwater, just before the bath has filled to the desired depth, pouring it slowly under the hot water tap so the oil disperses through the water.

▼ SLOWLY ADD DILUTED OIL TO BATHWATER.

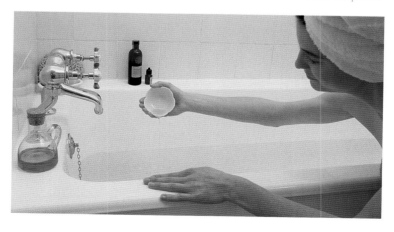

Mixing and storing essential oils

When essential oils are used for aromatherapy massage, different oils are combined to increase their therapeutic effect. Once you have mixed your oils, store and use them immediately, as they are perishable.

Aromatic essential oils may be used in a number of ways to maintain and restore health, and to improve our quality of life with their scents. Essential oils are concentrated substances and as such they need to be diluted for safety and optimum effect.

The ratio of essential oil to carrier oil varies, but, as a rule, ten drops of essential oil in 20ml/4tsp carrier oil is enough for a body massage. This gives a standard 2.5 per cent dilution, recommended for most uses.

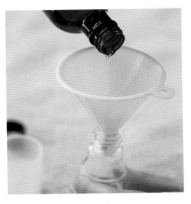

▲ USE A FUNNEL TO AVOID SPILLAGE.

Experiment with different types of vegetable oil to find the ideal blend for your massage style. Add a teaspoonful of another vegetable oil as well as the essential oils for an exotic and personal mixture.

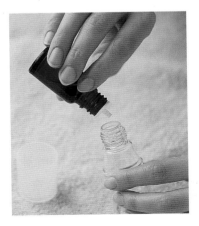

◀ BLEND OILS ONE DROP AT A TIME.

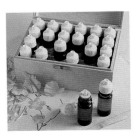

▶ STORE OILS IN DARK BOTTLES.

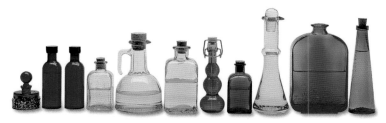

To blend essential oils for massage, first pour the vegetable oil into a blending bowl. Then add the essential oil a drop at a time and stir gently with a cocktail stick (toothpick) to blend. Test the fragrance before beginning, as it may need adjusting.

Essential oils are liable to deteriorate through the action of sunlight, so should be stored in a cool, dark place and away from direct heat. They should always be bought in dark-coloured glass

▲ STORE CARRIER OILS CAREFULLY TO ENSURE THEIR FRESHNESS.

bottles with a stopper that dispenses them a drop at a time. Only blend a small quantity of oils at a time to prevent the mixture deteriorating. Citrus oils tend to go off more quickly than other oils, so it is best to buy them in small amounts as you need them.

▼ USE AROMATHERAPY BLENDS IMMEDIATELY OR STORE IN SEALED BOTTLES AS ESSENTIAL OILS EVAPORATE QUICKLY.

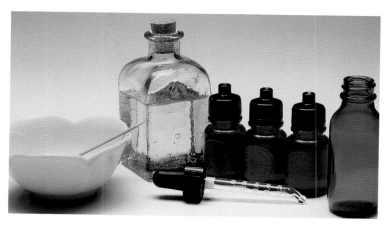

Citrus oils

Many citrus fruits yield essential oils, and they tend to have similar properties. In general they are refreshing, stimulating oils, good for the morning bath, leaving you feeling cleansed and alive.

ORANGES

The bitter, or Seville, orange is the source of three different oils, from the fruit, the blossom (also known as neroli) and the leaf (also called petitgrain). All have a mellow, warming and soothing effect, and are a good tonic and mood lifter, raising the libido.

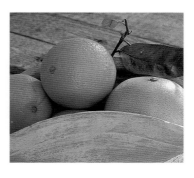

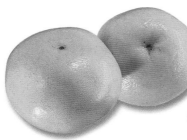

GRAPEFRUIT

This uplifting oil, taken from the fruit's fresh peel, helps to digest fatty foods, and combat cellulite and congested pores. It also soothes headaches and nervous exhaustion.

NEROLI

This oil is particularly effective for nervous tension, headaches, insomnia and other stress-related conditions. It can also be used to create a feeling of peace and is useful during times of anxiety, panic, hysteria or shock and fear. It can also help in the development of self-esteem and self-love.

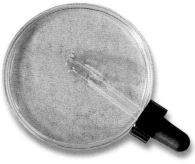

LIMES

Oil of lime is good for stimulating a sluggish system and may be used when a tonic is needed, in massage or in the bath.

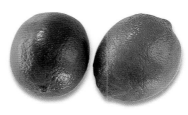

MANDARINS

Refreshing and cleansing, this sweetly scented oil is especially good for skin problems such as acne. It also helps digestion, soothing heartburn and nausea.

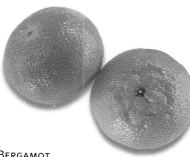

BERGAMOT

The peel of the ripe fruit yields an oil that is mild and gentle. It is the most effective antidepressant oil of all, best used at the start of the day. The oil can be used on a burner for lifting the atmosphere. Do not use on the skin in bright sunlight, as it can cause irritation.

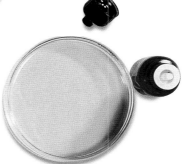

LEMONS

Possibly the most cleansing and antiseptic of the citrus oils, lemon oil is useful for boosting the immune and respiratory systems, and for use in skin care. It can also refresh and clarify thoughts, preventing feelings of bitterness or anger about life's injustices.

Shrub and vine oils

Essential oils can be extracted from many different parts of plants. Rose and jasmine oils are obtained from the flowers, the oil of black pepper comes from the fruit of a tropical vine, and geranium oil is taken from the plant's leaves.

JASMINE

One of the most wonderful aromas, jasmine has a relaxing, euphoric effect, and can lift the mood when there is debility, depression and general listlessness. Use in the bath or in massage oils.

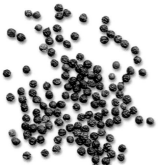

BLACK PEPPER

The essential oil of black pepper is warming and comforting and can often add mysterious depth to a blend. It is particularly effective for treating muscular aches and pains, and relieving colds and fevers.

GERANIUM

Rose-scented geranium oil is obtained from the shrub's leaves. It has a refreshing antidepressant quality, which is good for nervous tension and exhaustion, and can combine a blend to make a more harmonious scent.

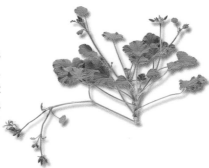

LAVENDER

Extracted from lavender flowers, this oil is the most versatile of all essential oils. It has been used for centuries to bring freshness and fragrance to the home, and as a remedy for stress-related ailments.

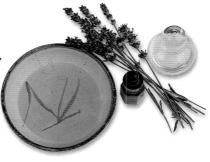

JUNIPER

Good for strengthening the spirits and purifying the atmosphere, this oil is obtained from juniper berries. Its most important use is as a detoxifier, but it is also effective for cystitis, cellulite, water retention, and absence of or painful menstrual periods.

ROSE

Probably the most famous of all oils, rose is good for sedating, calming and as an effective anti-inflammatory. Use in the bath or add to a base massage oil to soothe muscular and nervous tension.

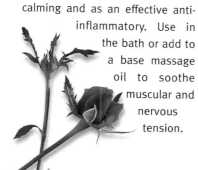

ROSEMARY

This stimulating oil, taken from the plant's leaves, has been used for centuries to help relieve nervous exhaustion, tension headaches and migraines. It improves circulation to the brain, and is an excellent oil for mental fatigue and debility. It is also an effective remedy for fluid retention.

Herb and spice oils

The essential oils of many herbs and spices contain powerful healing properties, which should be enjoyed but also respected. Nature provides an abundance of therapeutic compounds to help restore health and vitality.

CLARY SAGE

This essential oil, taken from the leaves, gives a euphoric uplift to the brain; be careful how much you use, however, as it can leave you feeling very intoxicated! Its relaxing and antidepressant qualities have contributed to its reputation as an aphrodisiac.

PEPPERMINT

The plant's leaves are used to produce this oil which is a classic ingredient in inhalations for relieving catarrh. Peppermint's analgesic and antispasmodic effects make it very useful for rubbing onto the temples to ease tension headaches; ideally dilute a drop in a little base cream or oil before applying.

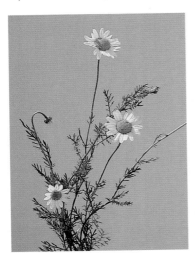

CHAMOMILE

The flowering parts of Roman and German chamomile are used to obtain essential oils with very similar properties. Chamomile oil is relaxing and antispasmodic, and helps to relieve tension headaches, nervous digestive problems and insomnia. It is also a gentle sedative oil for people who are highly strung and over-enthusiastic.

MARJORAM

Obtained from marjoram leaves, this oil has a calming and warming effect, and is good for both cold muscles and for cold and tense people who might also suffer from headaches, migraines or insomnia.

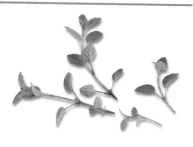

GINGER

Extracted from the ginger root, this oil is known for its warm and comforting nature. It is a balancing oil and counteracts ailments caused by dampness, being particularly effective for muscular aches and pains, catarrh and other symptoms of coughs and colds.

NUTMEG

With its warming, stimulating and euphoric effects, this oil, taken from the fruit of the nutmeg tree, aids poor circulation, muscular aches, sluggish digestion, loss of appetite and the early stages of a cold. It can also be comforting to those who feel emotionally isolated.

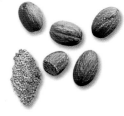

PALMAROSA

Taken from the leaves of this herbaceous plant, palmarosa is a gentle and comforting oil. It is particularly effective for acne, dermatitis, scars, sores and other skin inflammations, as well as weak digestion, headaches and nervous exhaustion.

Tree oils

Oils can be obtained from a variety of trees; with some, for example, cedarwood, the oil is extracted by steam distillation from the wood, whereas with others, such as ylang ylang, the oils come from the flowers.

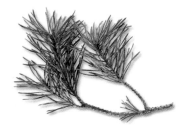

Pine
The pine oil used in aromatherapy generally comes from the Scots pine. It helps to clear the air passages when used as an inhalation, and is also good for relieving fatigue. Tired, aching muscles can be eased with massage using diluted pine oil.

Eucalyptus
Extracted from eucalyptus leaves, this is one of the finest oils for respiratory complaints, eucalyptus is found in most commercial inhalants. Well diluted in a base vegetable oil, eucalyptus can be applied to the forehead to help relieve a hot, tense headache linked with tiredness.

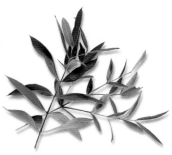

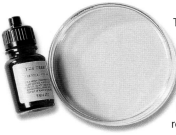

Tea tree
Vigorous and revitalizing, tea tree oil is effective in fighting infectious organisms. It is also a powerful immune stimulant, increasing the body's ability to respond to these organisms.

Sandalwood

Probably the oldest perfume in history, sandalwood has been used for 4,000 years. It has a heavy scent, and often appeals to men as much as to women. It has a relaxing, antidepressant effect on the nervous system, and where depression causes sexual problems, sandalwood can be used as a genuine aphrodisiac.

Cedarwood

Thought to be one of the earliest known essential oils, cedarwood oil is effective for long-standing complaints rather than acute ones, such as acne, dandruff, arthritis, rheumatism, bronchitis and chest infections. This uplifting oil is useful for treating lack of confidence or fearfulness, and can help to eliminate mental stagnation. Its relaxing and soothing properties can be a good aid to meditation. Cedarwood is also an aphrodisiac.

Cypress

With a rich scent similar to the scent of pine needles, cypress oil is useful for treating conditions that cause excess fluids, such as diarrhoea, water retention and watery colds. The oil, extracted from the tree's cones, can be uplifting in cases of sadness or self-pity, and can help to soothe anger.

Ylang ylang

The flowers of this tropical tree, native to Indonesia, produce an intensely sweet essential oil that has a sedative yet antidepressant action. It is good for many symptoms of excessive tension, such as insomnia, panic attacks, anxiety and depression.

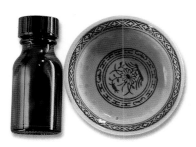

Aromatherapy massage

Massage is a wonderful way to use essential oils, suitably diluted in a good base oil, for your partner or family. Use soft, thick towels to cover areas of the body you are not massaging, and make sure that the room is warm.

Anyone will benefit from regular massage as it eases tense muscles and also helps us feel warm and relaxed. Although quite different and inevitably limited, self-massage is also an excellent way to help yourself relax and can help clear tension headaches and ease a stiff neck and shoulders.

Ideally, massage should be carried out just before a bath or when you can lie down in a warm place. Suitable base oils for massage include sweet almond oil (probably the most versatile and useful), grapeseed, safflower, soya (a bit thicker and stickier), coconut and even sunflower. For very dry skins, a small amount of jojoba, avocado or wheatgerm oils (except in cases of wheat allergy) may be added. Essential

▼ THE NURTURING TOUCH OF MASSAGE IS ENHANCED BY THE AROMA OF ESSENTIAL OILS.

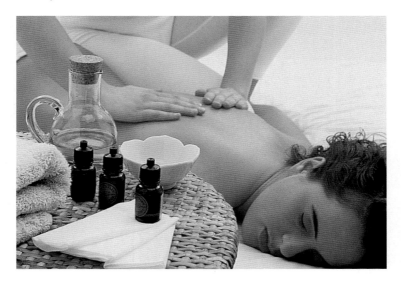

oils may be blended at a dilution of 1 per cent, or one drop per 5ml/1tsp base oil; this may sometimes by increased to 2 per cent, but take care that no skin reactions occur with any oil.

If someone has sensitive skin or suffers from allergies, try massaging with one drop of essential oil per 20ml/4tsp base oil to test for any reaction. Seek medical advice before massaging a pregnant woman.

Prepare for massage by playing some soft music, lowering the lights or lighting candles and ensure your partner is lying comfortably on the floor with a clean towel spread beneath them.

CAUTION

If your partner has sensitive skin or suffers from allergies, massage with just one drop of essential oil per 20ml/4 tsp base oil at first to test for any reaction. Always seek medical advice before massaging a pregnant woman.

The oil for the massage, blended with essential oil, should be poured into a small, clean bowl from where you can take more oil from time to time without disturbing the rhythm of the massage. It is always a good idea to stand the bowl of oil on a towel in order to protect the underlying surface from spills.

MIXING OILS FOR MASSAGE

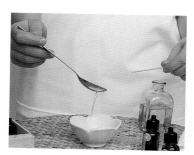

1 Pour about 10ml/2tsp of your chosen vegetable oil into a blending bowl.

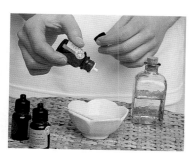

2 Add the essential oil, one drop at a time. Mix with a clean dry cocktail stick or toothpick.

Aromatherapy blends

A selection of blends of essential oils for everyday circumstances is given below. These few suggestions are to be used as a guide. If you already have a favourite blend, there is no reason why you should not use it.

Choose up to four essential oils to make an appropriate blend. Mix with a carrier or base oil.

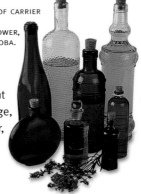

▶ THE VARIETY OF CARRIER OILS INCLUDES ALMOND, SUNFLOWER, SESAME AND JOJOBA.

TO AID RELAXATION

For a relaxing massage choose three or four oils from the following list: bergamot, clary sage, lavender, sandalwood and German chamomile. Inlcude one of the citrus oils, to add an uplifting note to the blend.

REMEDY FOR OVER-INDULGENCE

A gentle massage using three or four of any of the following oils may help to restore balance following an over-indulgent period: orange, black pepper, geranium, juniper and ginger.

▼ CAREFULLY MEASURE OUT THE CORRECT QUANTITY OF BASE OIL.

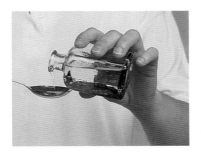

TO DISPEL GLOOM

Try making a blend of three or four of the following essential oils: black pepper, cypress, eucalyptus, ginger, grapefruit, jasmine, juniper, lemon, nutmeg, peppermint, rosemary and tea tree.

FOR STIFF MUSCLES

Everyone suffers from minor muscular aches and pains from time to time. Warming essential oils are the most helpful for stiff muscles. You can choose from any of the following: black pepper, ginger, clary sage, eucalyptus,

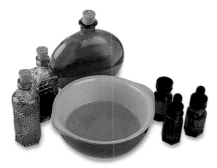

◄ MIX YOUR BLEND OF ESSENTIAL OILS WITH A CARRIER, OR BASE, OIL IN A SMALL BOWL READY FOR USE.

peppermint, grapefruit, jasmine, juniper, lavender, lemon, orange, marjoram and nutmeg.

AN APHRODISIAC BLEND

Tension, anxiety, worry, depression – all these can affect your sexual energy. This can result in a downward spiral of anxiety about sex, and cause reduced enjoyment. Try to take time out of your hectic life to spend time together with your partner and have fun: add to your sensual pleasure with an intimate massage session, using one of these blends to release tensions and allow your natural sexual energy to respond.

Use a blend that appeals to you both – either five drops rose and five drops sandalwood or four drops jasmine and four drops ylang ylang and include in a massage oil. Use gentle, stroking movements all over the back, buttocks, legs and front.

SENSUAL MASSAGE

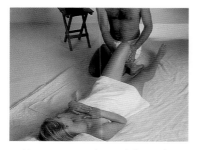

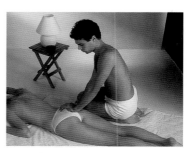

1 Use rose and sandalwood, or jasmine and ylang ylang oil to massage gently all over the body.

2 Apply a firmer pressure when massaging large muscles such as the buttocks.

aromatherapy blends **135**

Massage strokes

Massage techniques are relatively simple to learn. They range from a gentle, stroking action that relaxes the body to a more vigorous kneading, pummelling or hacking motion to stimulate and energize the system.

PETRISSAGE

Kneading or petrissage movements stimulate the circulation and encourage the drainage of toxins. The basic kneading action is similar to kneading dough.

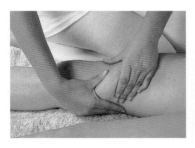

1 Grasp the flesh between fingers and thumb and push it towards the other hand. As you release the first hand, your second hand grasps the flesh and pushes it back towards the first hand. It is a continuous action, alternating the hands to squeeze and release.

WRINGING

Like petrissage, wringing relies on the action of one hand pushing against the other.

1 Place your right hand, palm facing downwards, over the hip opposite to you and cup your left hand over the hip closest to you. Slide your hands towards each other with enough pressure to lift and roll the flesh on the sides of the body.

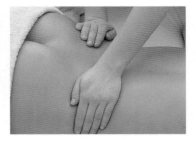

2 Decrease the pressure as you stroke across the back to your original position, hands passing each other to the opposite sides of the body. Without stopping, begin to slide them back again. Stroke your hands back and forth continuously while you wring up and down the lower back. The dual action of the hands creates a powerful squeezing motion.

Friction

Use friction techniques, such as pressure and knuckling, to work on specific areas of muscular tightness. Pressure techniques are less painful when performed along the direction of the muscle fibres.

1 To apply static pressure, press firmly into the muscle with the thumbs. Lean into the movement with the body, slowly deepening the pressure and then release.

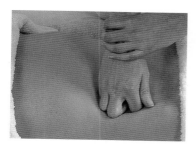

2 To release tension up the sides of the spine, use the knuckles in a loosely clenched fist on either side of the spine to produce rippling, circular movements.

CAUTION
Do not use tapotement on bony areas of the body. Never apply pressure on or below broken or varicose veins.

Tapotement

These movements are fast and stimulating, improving the circulation, and toning the skin and muscles. They are useful for working on fleshy areas of the body. Remember to keep your hands and wrists relaxed.

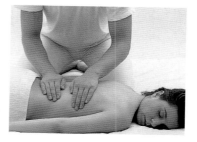

1 Cup the hands and make a brisk cupping action against a fleshy area, alternating the hands.

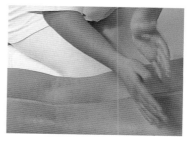

2 Use the outer edge of the palm and a chopping or hacking motion with alternate hands. Work rhythmically and rapidly.

Facial massage

A face massage dissolves anxiety and stress, eases away headaches, and enhances relaxation. Let your strokes be firm but gentle, following the natural symmetry of the bone structure and facial features.

Receiving a face massage is a wonderful way to finish a body massage, or combined with the chest, neck and head strokes, it can be a deeply satisfying and effective session in its own right.

When giving your partner a face massage, you should try to focus your total attention on to your hands and fingers so that each touch is feather like and made with great sensitivity.

GENTLE STROKES

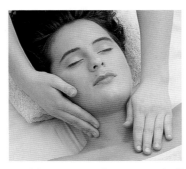

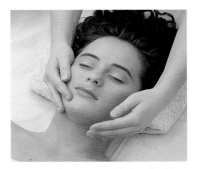

1 Add a very small amount of oil to your hands to ensure a smooth glide over the skin. Then softly stroke your hands, one following the other, up over the chest, neck and sides of the face, moulding them to the natural contours of the face.

2 A gentle caress of the jawline will be comforting to your partner. With slightly cupped hands, stroke one hand after the other in alternating movements along both sides of the face. Move from the point of the chin round towards the ears.

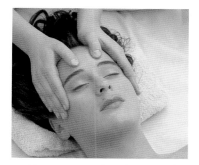

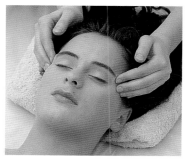

1 Place your thumbs on the forehead, while your hands cradle the face. Draw the thumbs towards the side, finishing with a sweep around the temples.

2 Keeping your hands relaxed and cupped, use your fingertips to stroke the temples very softly several times in a clockwise circular movement.

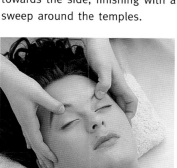

3 The hollows under the ridge of the brow are sinus passages. Gentle pressure on these points can help to release tension headaches. Press sensitively up under the ridge, on one spot at a time, with your thumb pads.

TIP
Choose the blend of oils for the massage according to your partner's needs: if they are tense and over-tired, a relaxing blend of lavender, chamomile and clary sage oils could be helpful; if they need to be revitalized, geranium and bergamot oils will give them an energizing boost.

Continue to hold the pressure under the ridge for a count of five before releasing it slowly. Move from the inner to the outer edge of the eyebrows.

CIRCLING THE CHEEKBONES

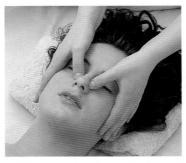

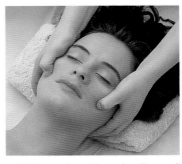

1 Slip your thumbs each side of the bridge of the nose, while wrapping your hands against the sides of the cheeks. Slide both thumbs down each side of the nose to the edge of the nostrils.

2 Without breaking the flow of motion, draw your thumb pads out under the cheekbones, indenting them slightly up under the ridge of the bone.

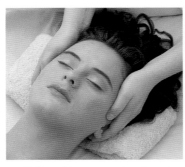

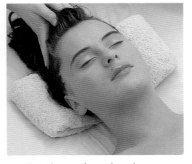

3 Soften the pressure in your thumbs as they reach the sides of the face, and begin to pull both hands soothingly up towards the top of the head.

4 Continue by drawing your hands and fingers out through the head and hair until they pull away from the body. Bring your hands back to the first position of the stroke. Repeat twice.

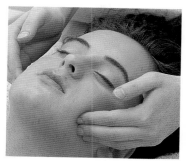

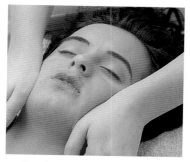

1 Relax your hands and sink your fingertips into the cheek muscles. Rotate them, counter-clockwise, several times on one area before moving to the next fleshy area.

2 Gently press and rotate the heels of your hands in continuous but alternate movements on the cheeks to increase suppleness and to loosen the muscles surrounding the mouth.

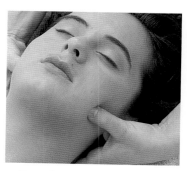

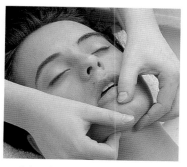

3 To reduce tension in the jaw muscles, slip your fingers behind the neck, and sink your thumbs into the muscle before rotating them on one spot at a time.

4 Grip the jaw bone with your fingers and use your thumbs to stroke over the chin in small circles, applying more pressure on the down and outward slide.

Self-massage

Give yourself a real treat with these simple self-massage techniques. Choose an appropriate blend of essential oils, and add at 1 per cent dilution to a base oil such as sweet almond. Oil your hands before spreading it on to your skin.

Self-massage is an excellent way to help yourself relax and can help clear tension headaches and ease a stiff neck and shoulders. There is an undoubted sensuality about massage, the feel of oil on the skin and the gradual easing of tension, so enjoy this opportunity to pamper yourself. The benefit is not only from the gentle application of massage oil but also from the time taken to care for yourself and your needs.

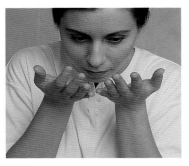

▲ DEPENDING ON THE OIL USED, THE AROMA OF AN ESSENTIAL OIL MASSAGE CAN HELP TO RELAX AND EASE TENSION OR UPLIFT YOUR MIND AND ENERGIZE YOUR BODY.

THE FACE

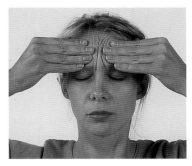

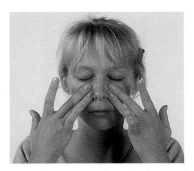

1 Use small circling movements with the fingers, over the forehead, temples and cheeks.

2 Work across the cheeks and along each side of the nose, then out to the jaw line.

THE HANDS

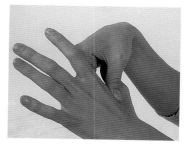

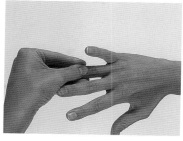

1 You can help to reduce any tension in your hands by firmly squeezing the fleshy area between each finger with the thumb and fingers of the other hand, rolling the flesh a little to give a kneading effect.

2 Squeeze and gently stretch each finger one after the other, working from the base of your finger out towards the tip. Now repeat this exercise on the other hand.

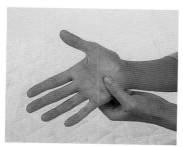

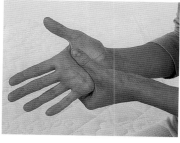

3 With a firm movement, knead the palm with the thumb of your other hand, making strong circular strokes. This squeezes and stretches taut, contracted muscles, and should be a fairly deep action.

4 Continue this kneading action as you work steadily across the palm of your hand, maintaining a firm pressure. Now repeat these movements on the other hand.

THE LEGS

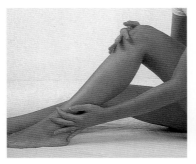 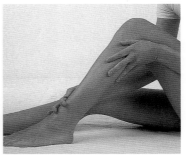

1 Sit with one leg bent, so that you can comfortably reach down as far as the ankle.

2 Sweep up the leg from ankle to knee, using alternate hands. This helps to move venous blood back towards the heart.

THE FEET

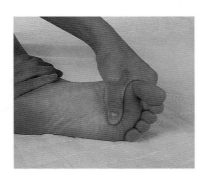

1 Sit so that you can comfortably reach a foot, and with quite a firm grip use small circular strokes all over the sole with your thumb. Pay special attention to the arch of the foot, stretching along the line of the arch with your thumb.

THE ARMS

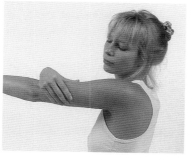 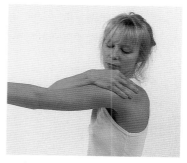

1 Grip your arm at the wrist and squeeze. Repeat this action up the length of the arm.

2 Continue up the arm to the shoulder. Switch arms and repeat the exercise.

THE SHOULDERS

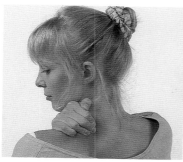 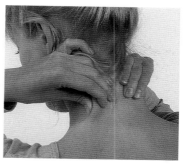

1 Firmly grip your shoulder and use a squeezing motion to loosen the tension, moving along the shoulder several times. Repeat on the other side.

2 Work up as far as the base of the skull, squeezing the neck muscles with your fingertips, and work your way down again.

Massage with a partner

One of the best ways to remove stress and tension from your partner is by massage. The effects of the following simple massage movements can be enhanced greatly by adding essential oils at 1 per cent dilution to the base oil.

When using essential oils in massage with a partner, you are sharing the therapeutic effect, so choose a blend that you both like.

Prepare the massage space beforehand so that it is warm and relaxing. Ensure that your partner is lying comfortably: use cushions or pillows for support if necessary, and cover them with towels, if needed, for warmth. Always warm the oil in your hands before applying it to the skin.

For a relaxing massage, begin with the back, move to the face, then finish with the arms and feet. This should ease headaches and tension and promote a feeling of deep and utter relaxation. Always use gentle strokes.

THE BACK

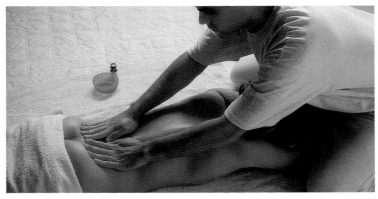

Place your hands on either side of the spine, on the line of muscles that run down the back. Move down the back using a slow gliding motion. Take your hands further out to the side and glide back up towards the shoulders, before repeating this stroke.

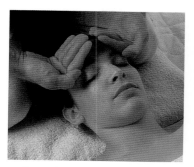

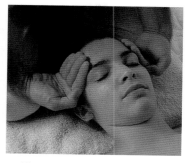

1 Smooth across the forehead with the back of your hands. Start the stroking motion at the centre of the forehead and move towards the temples.

2 These movements can often ease a headache, especially when it is still at an early stage, and are very calming.

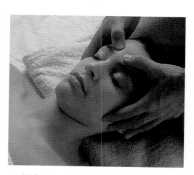

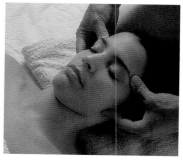

3 Using your thumbs or fingers, work steadily over the forehead in small circles, moving out over the temples to help to ease tight, tense muscles.

4 Continue this movement down the temples to the jaw line for an even greater relaxing effect. Use firm pressure, squeezing the skin with each circle.

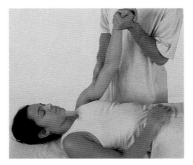

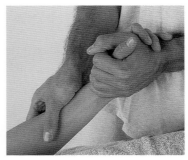

1 Support your partner's arm, raising it into the air and squeeze down the whole length of the arm with your thumb and fingers to encourage the blood and lymph to flow back towards the heart.

2 Let the upper arm rest on the floor, then work on the forearm with stroking movements from the wrist to the elbow – you may need to swap your hands to work around each side of the arm.

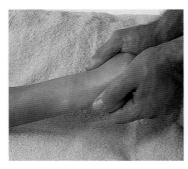

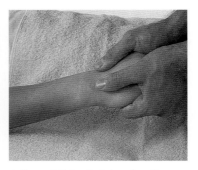

3 To help relieve tension from your partner's hands, hold one hand, palm down, in your hands and apply a steady stretching motion over the back of the hand.

4 Repeat this stretch a few times, with a firm but comfortable pressure on the hand. Repeat all these movements on the other arm and hand.

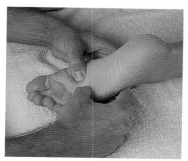

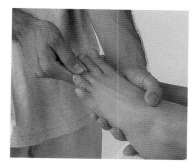

1 Use your thumbs to press firmly in small circles all over the sole. Keep the movements slow and deep, and finish with long lines running from the toes to the heel.

2 Hold one of the toes and give a squeeze and pulling action. Repeat for all the toes.

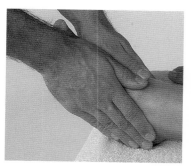

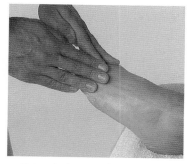

3 Smooth all the way up and down the upper side of the foot with both hands.

4 Extend the stroking from the ankle to the toes, then return to the centre; smooth back up the foot. Repeat on the other foot.

Baby massage

All babies thrive on being cuddled, touched, and massaged. Skin-to-skin contact is essential to the nurturing of infants, helping them to bond with their parents, and to develop emotional and physical health.

SOOTHING AND FEATHERING

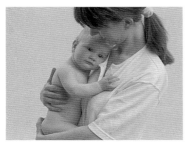

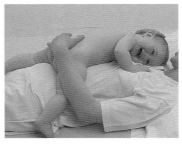

1 Hold your baby close to you, so they can feel the warmth of your body, the beat of your heart, and the rhythm of your breathing, enabling them to be comforted.

2 Babies love to lie against the softness of your body. Soothe them by placing one hand over the base of the spine, while gently stroking the head.

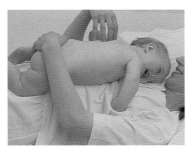

3 Running your fingertips up and down your baby's back will make them giggle as the feather-like touches brush their delicate skin.

OILS FOR BABIES AND YOUNGSTERS

Choose from the following essential oils:

Newborn infants: chamomile, geranium, lavender, mandarin and eucalyptus.

Infants 2–6 months old: as above plus neroli and peppermint.

Infants 6–12 months old: as above plus grapefruit, palmarosa and tea tree.

FLEXING AND WIGGLING

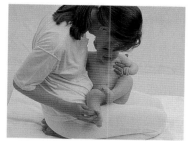

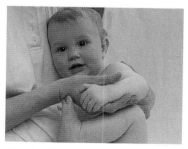

1 Your baby will enjoy this game of passive movements. Bend the knee towards the body and then straighten out the leg. Carry out the same action on the other leg. Repeat several times.

2 Babies never seem to lose interest in their fingers and toes; add to this fascination by wiggling and rotating the little joints one by one.

EFFLEURAGE

KNEADING AND SQUEEZING

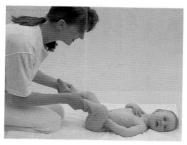

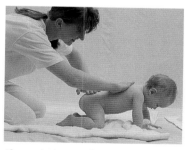

If your baby can keep still for long enough, you can rub nourishing oil into the skin while massaging. Soft effleurage strokes on the back, such as fanning and circles, will delight them.

Chubby little arms and legs are made for gentle squeezing and kneading. Press the limbs softly between your thumb and fingers.

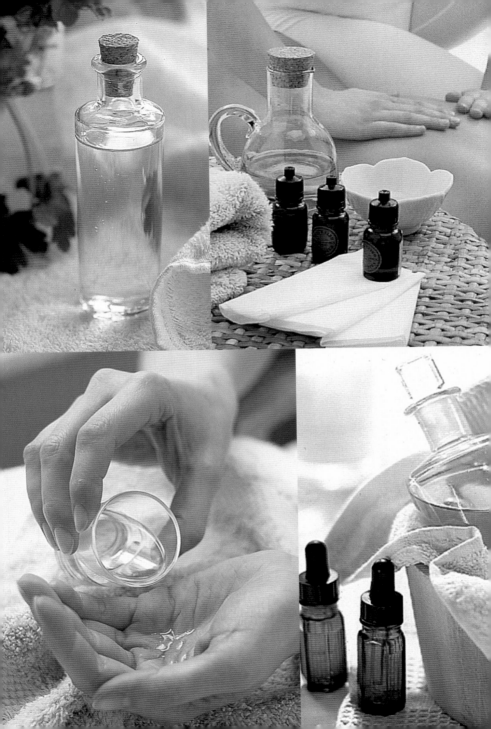

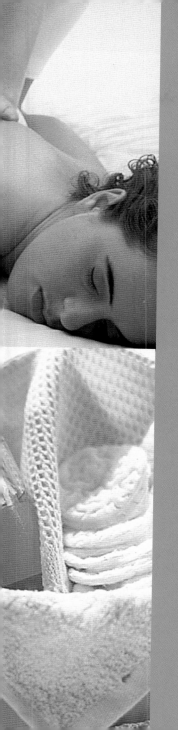

AROMATHERAPY
TREATMENTS

Now that you understand the properties of essential oils, and have learned how to blend them for use in aromatherapy massage, you can apply this knowledge to a wider range of home treatments for everyday complaints.

Aromatherapy works on every level to cleanse the body and calm the mind, and it can be used in response to issues such as stress, headache, poor digestion, low vitality, skin complaints, menstrual pains and muscular aches. In addition to massage therapies, try out inhalations, compresses, hair rinses and a range of pleasurable soaking remedies perfect for soothing the feet or whole body. These simple and effective treatments can easily be incorporated into a daily routine.

Energizers

There are unfortunately times in all our lives when we get depressed, whether due to a specific event or from chronic tiredness. As part of a programme of recuperation and restoring vitality, aromatherapy can be very effective.

UPLIFTING OILS

For a strong, but relatively short-lived effect, try four drops bergamot and two drops neroli in the bath, ideally in the morning. After the bath, gently pat the skin with a soft towel. Do not rub vigorously. A gentler effect, which can pervade the atmosphere all day long, is to use bergamot or neroli oils in an essential oil burner – probably just one drop of each oil at a time, repeating as needed.

INVIGORATING OILS

Chronic tension all too often leads to a feeling of exhaustion, when we just run out of steam. At these times we need a boost,

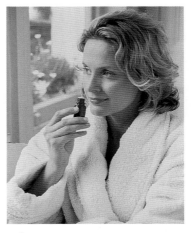

▲ ESSENTIAL OILS CAN PROVIDE AN INSTANT PICK-ME-UP.

and many oils have a tonic effect, restoring vitality without over-stimulating. As a group, citrus oils are good for this purpose, ranging from the soothing mandarin to the refreshing lemon oil.

Have a warm bath, with four drops mandarin and two drops orange or four drops neroli and two drops lemon. Alternatively, just add a couple of drops of

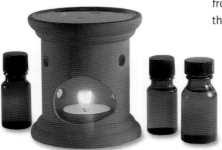

◀ VAPORIZED OILS CAN HAVE A VERY UPLIFTING EFFECT ON THE SPIRITS.

◀ LEMON OIL
REFRESHES AND
CLEARS THE MIND.

▶ ROSEMARY IS
USEFUL FOR MENTAL
FATIGUE OR LETHARGY.

any of these oils to a bowl of steaming water and gently inhale to help to lift tiredness and raise your spirits.

Steam inhalation is a valuable and simple way to receive the benefits of essential oils when time or circumstance prevents massage or a bath.

Revitalizing oils

In today's high pressure world, trying to juggle with too many demands leads nearly all of us to reach a state of "brain fag" at some point, when mental fatigue and exhaustion grind us to a halt.

Rather than reach for the coffee, or worse still alcohol, which may seem to relax but actually depresses the central nervous system, try using these revitalizing oils to give you an instant pick-me-up and make you feel more alert.

You can use one to two drops of rosemary or peppermint oil in a burner. Alternatively, add three drops rosemary and two drops peppermint to a bowl of steaming water, or use four drops of either oil on their own. Allow the oils to evaporate into the room.

▼ A STEAM INHALATION OF ESSENTIAL OILS CAN HELP TO UPLIFT YOUR SPIRITS.

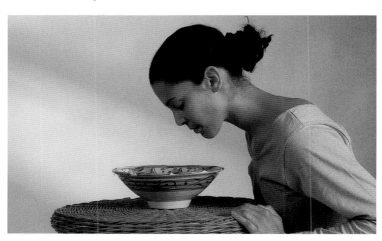

Inhalations

Colds and sinus problems may cause congestion, but we can also feel blocked up and unable to breathe freely through tension. Steam inhalations warm and moisten the membranes, and essential oils help to open the airways.

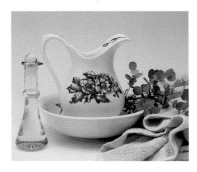

◀ A EUCALYPTUS STEAM INHALATION HELPS TO CLEAR CONGESTION.

CAUTION

If you have either high blood pressure or asthma you should seek medical advice before using steam, and in any case do not overdo an inhalation.

▼ INHALE THE STEAM DEEPLY.

For a stuffed-up feeling, maybe combined with tiredness, try using three drops eucalyptus and two drops peppermint oil in a bowl of steaming water.

For tension causing poor breathing, relax the airways with four drops lavender and three drops frankincense.

Steam inhalations are helpful for respiratory complaints. Use a total of ten drops for a strong medicinal effect, in cases of colds and chestiness, or just five drops for a gentler relaxing effect. Inhale the steam deeply while holding a towel over your head to slow down the rate of oil evaporation.

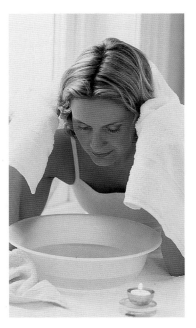

Sprains and swellings

Hot or cold compresses are excellent ways to use oils for problems such as sprains and muscular aches. To make a compress, add essential oils to iced or hot water and soak a pad in it before placing on the affected area.

Cold compresses are suitable for use on acute injuries such as a strain or sprain, with swelling or bruising. For older injuries, for chronic muscle aches such as backache and menstrual pain, and for arthritic or rheumatic pain, a hot compress may be more useful.

The ideal oil for a cold compress is lavender, which is useful in many first-aid situations. Use four drops to a bowl of iced water. Keep the pad on for at least 20 minutes. Raise the affected limb if a swelling occurs.

For muscular aches, try using two drops of both rosemary and marjoram in a bowl of hot water. Apply for 30 minutes.

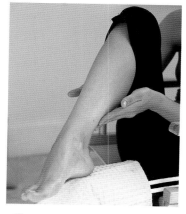

▲ STRAINS MAY OCCUR AS A RESULT OF FAILING TO WARM UP BEFORE EXERCISE.

▼ A COLD COMPRESS IS GOOD FOR SOOTHING STRAINS AND SPRAINS.

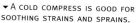

▼ COMPRESSES CAN STIMULATE CIRCULATION.

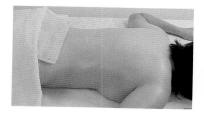

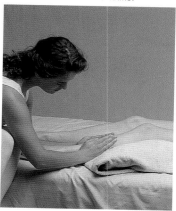

Backache relievers

So often people carry around their tensions in the form of a stiff, aching or knotted back. Symptoms can range from tight shoulders to lower backache. The best way of using oils to relieve backache is in massage of the taut muscles.

When massaging your partner's back to relieve pain, long sweeping strokes along the length of the back and a deep kneading action with the hands will loosen areas of muscle spasm, while the aromatic essential oils will work their magic and relax tension.

Two essential oil blends that will help to work on deeper tensions and knotted muscles are three drops pine and three drops rosemary oil, or four drops lavender used with three drops marjoram oil mixed with the base oil. The oil for the massage should be poured into a small, clean bowl close to hand, from where you can take more oil from time to time as you need it without disturbing the rhythm of the massage.

▸ PENETRATING ROSEMARY OIL
IS PARTICULARLY BENEFICIAL
FOR RELIEVING MUSCULAR ACHES.

RELAXING TENSE BACKS

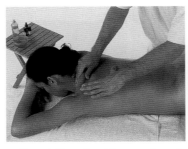

1 Knead the shoulders and neck to ease stiff, tense muscles.

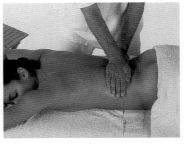

2 Apply steady, sweeping movements down the back with your hands. Finally, stroke firmly down the back with both hands.

Muscular ache relievers

When you are under stress for any length of time, your body stays permanently tense. This can make any or all of your muscles ache and feel tired or heavy. Massage with a blend of essential oils will begin to relieve symptoms.

Gentle but firm massage is a wonderful reviver of tired, tender or tense muscles, especially when the aches are smoothed away with a fragrant oil. As the massage movements start to work on the aching muscles, the oils are being absorbed and get to work on inner tension too.

For the best effect, use a blend of three drops pine, three drops marjoram and two drops juniper oil for a variety of soothing massage strokes. Other warming oils that help to relieve aching muscles include: black pepper, clary sage, eucalyptus, ginger, grapefruit, jasmine, lavender, lemon, peppermint, orange, nutmeg and rosemary. You can also try experimenting with different blends of essential oils to discover which ones suit you best.

▶ A MASSAGE WITH PINE OIL IS IDEAL FOR INVIGORATING TIRED MUSCLES.

MASSAGING ACHING BACK MUSCLES

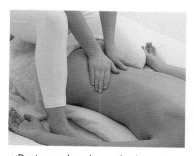

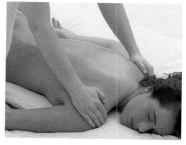

1 Rest your hands on the lower back on either side of the spine. Lean your weight into your hands and stroke firmly up the back. Mould your hands to the body as you go.

2 As your hands reach the top of your partner's back, fan them gently out towards the shoulders using a smooth, flowing motion.

Headache soothers

 Tension headaches are a common feature in many people's lives, and may come from long hours at the computer or even longer hours with small children! Whatever the cause, gentle massage can help.

To relieve headaches, gentle massage of the temples and forehead at the earliest moment can help to stop headaches from getting a tight grip. Another option is the application of a warm compress soaked in hot water blended with essential oils.

If your head feels hot, try using an oil with four drops of peppermint. If warmth feels helpful, then you could try applying six drops of lavender oil. Another option for soothing a headache caused by congestion or tension is to use four drops of chamomile oil.

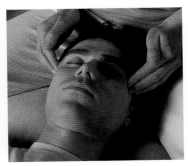

RELIEVING A HEADACHE

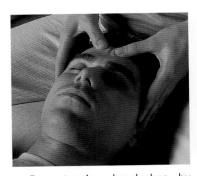

1 Ease tension headaches by massaging aromatherapy oils into the forehead. With your thumbs, use steady but gentle pressure to stroke the forehead.

2 Gently massage the temples with your fingers, using slow rotating movements, in order to ease aches and pains caused by too much stress and tension.

◀ MARJORAM

▶ CLARY SAGE

One of the most complex of health problems, migraines are nature's way of shutting our systems down when life has been too demanding. The triggers that spark off a migraine attack are highly individual and professional treatment is really needed to try to understand the causes for each person.

At the first sign of a migraine, try using a blend of two drops rosemary, one drop marjoram and one drop clary sage, diluted in a base oil and gently massaged into the forehead and temples. Alternatively, use a drop of each essential oil in a bowl of warm water and apply a warm compress to the forehead.

ALLEVIATING A MIGRAINE

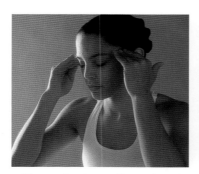

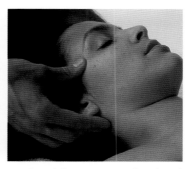

1 Many migraine sufferers have a heightened sense of smell at the onset of the attack and may find any aroma intolerable, so use oils sparingly. For self-help, gently massage the temples with small circling movements.

2 Receiving a gentle head massage from a partner allows you to lie back and relax your body completely and can therefore be even more effective than a self-massage at soothing the pain.

Menstrual pain easers

Painful periods can be due to several factors, but tension will certainly add to muscle spasm and cramping pains. If there is no organic or structural cause of the discomfort, try using essential oils as a hot compress or in the bath.

Some essential oils have a reputation for improving the menstrual cycle in ways other than as a compress or added to a hot bath; seek advice from a professional aromatherapist for longer-term treatments.

For a hot compress, soak a pad in hot water mixed with one drop each of rose, geranium and clary sage essential oils. Apply the compress over the lower abdomen to relieve menstrual pain. Alternatively, a fairly hot bath with three drops of rose, three drops of geranium and two drops of clary sage oil will quickly relax the cramped or aching muscles.

▲ ROSE

▼ A HOT BATH WITH OILS IS RELAXING.

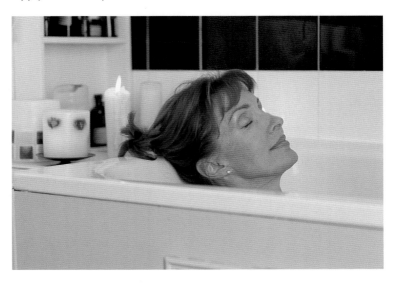

For many women the days leading up to a period can be fraught with mood swings, irritability and other symptoms. Professional treatment may be needed for full assistance; however, you could try this blend of essential oils if before each period you feel very tense and critical of those around you, or you just want to devour a box of chocolates!

Add three drops rose, three drops jasmine and two drops clary sage essential oil to a hot bath and lie back, allowing the aroma to soothe you, and letting the warm water soak away any tension in your body. Alternatively, you could try using this mixture in a massage oil and rub it gently into your lower abdomen for a soothing and relaxing effect.

▶ JASMINE

PREMENSTRUAL TENSION SOOTHER

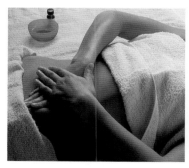

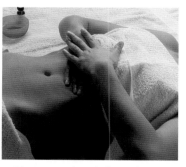

1 Slowly and firmly massage the lower abdomen with your hands. Close your eyes and continue the massage until you feel relaxed.

2 Move your hands in a clockwise direction, working up towards the chest; try to remain relaxed during this time so that the tension drains away.

Settling the stomach

Nervousness often results in an upset stomach. It has been said that our digestive organs also digest stress, and can end up storing emotions, causing discomfort and indigestion. The key is to let our bodies release anxieties.

Aromatherapy can help a great deal to achieve relaxation and calmness, allowing our bodies to release stress which may affect the digestive organs. One of the easiest ways to use oils in this context is to make a hot compress and place it over the abdomen, keeping the area warm for up to ten minutes.

To make the hot compress, add either two drops orange and three drops peppermint oil to a bowl of hot water, or you can use three drops chamomile and two drops orange essential oils. Soak a flannel in the scented water, wring it out, and apply it over the abdomen as directed above. The heat from the compress will soothe away stress and tension, and relax the abdominal muscles. Use the compress as often as necessary for relief, ensuring the flannel remains hot.

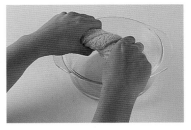

▲ SOAK A FLANNEL IN HOT WATER.

▼ LAY THE COMPRESS OVER THE ABDOMEN.

▼ SOOTHING PEPPERMINT TEA.

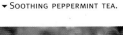

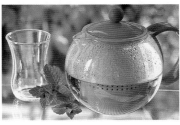

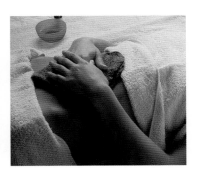

Travel calmers

It is said that travel broadens the mind; unfortunately, for some people it contracts the mind into a series of worries. Is this plane safe? Will I be sick? Try one of the following essential oils to calm the mind and stomach.

Inhaling essential oils while travelling allows you to enjoy the anticipation of new horizons without being stressed by how to reach them. The simplest way for you to use essential oils when travelling is to put a couple of drops onto a tissue or handkerchief, and to inhale them when you have need. Useful aromatherapy

◄ PEPPERMINT

▶ MANDARINS

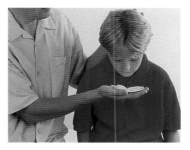

oils for this purpose include peppermint, mandarin and neroli. In addition to helping overcome travel sickness, peppermint is also useful for muscular aches and pains, nausea and colds. Mandarin oil has an uplifting effect and is also a good oil to use for treating restlessness and nervous tension. Likewise, neroli oil is useful during times of anxiety.

CALMING OILS

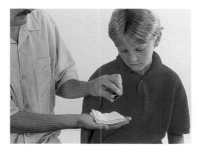

1 Put a couple of drops of aromatherapy oil onto a tissue or folded handkerchief.

2 Hold the tissue under the nose and lean the head slightly forwards. Inhale. Repeat as necessary throughout the journey.

Hair care

These days there is a bewildering range of products available for every type of hair. However, simpler treatments, which have been tried and trusted over many years, can also make your hair look wonderful.

Good hairdressers recommend a varied programme of hair care because consistently using one product can lead to build-up on the hair and scalp. Herbal hair rinses, shampoos and other treatments use natural ingredients which will leave your hair in really good condition.

The easiest way to make a herbal shampoo is to add 30–45ml/2–3tbsp of a strong herbal infusion to a gentle baby shampoo. Alternatively, you could

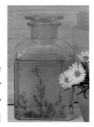

▶ STORE HERBAL HAIR RINSES IN GLASS BOTTLES.

add two to three drops of your favourite oil. For chamomile and orangeflower shampoo, mix 15ml/1tbsp chamomile infusion and five drops neroli essential oil into 60ml/4tbsp mild shampoo just before washing your hair.

HERBAL RINSE

A herbal rinse helps to keep the hair shiny and in good condition. When washing your hair, simply replace the last water rinse with a jugful of herbal rinse, mixed with water 50/50, and leave to dry. Chamomile and rosemary have been combined with vinegar and used in hair rinses for hundreds of years. The herbs enhance the colour of the hair and the vinegar is a wonderful scalp conditioner.

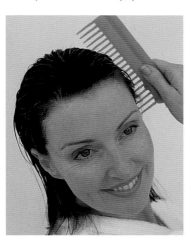

◀ COMB HAIR TREATMENT THROUGH HAIR.

Fair-hair rinse

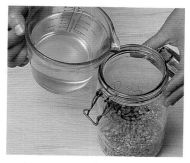

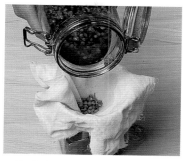

1 Measure 50g/2oz chamomile flowers in a jar. Pour 900ml/ 1½ pints boiled water over them.

2 Seal the jar and leave to stand overnight. Strain through muslin until the mixture is clear.

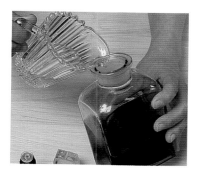

3 Add 50ml/2fl oz cider vinegar and five drops of chamomile essential oil. Store the mixture in a stoppered glass bottle in the fridge and use, within one week, as a final rinse whenever you wash your hair. The chamomile will enhance your hair's natural colour without bleaching.

Dark-hair rinse

This rinse uses the same basic ingredients as the fair-hair rinse but substitutes sprigs of fresh rosemary and rosemary oil for the chamomile flowers and oil. Pregnant women, however, should omit the rosemary essential oil.

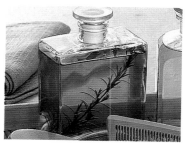

Skin care

When we become stressed, the small muscles close to the skin tend to contract. This can leave our skin undernourished with blood, and our complexion and skin tone suffer. Using essential oils can help counteract this.

Tense skin is frequently much drier than normal skin, and probably the best way to use essential oils is to mix them into your favourite skin cream. Obviously, this is best if the skin cream is originally unperfumed.

To make a reviving skin tonic, add three drops sandalwood and three drops rose oil, or four drops neroli and two drops rose oil to a 25g/1oz pot of skin cream. Mix together and apply to the skin.

To make a fragrant rose lotion which is excellent for all skin types, mix 175ml/6fl oz unscented

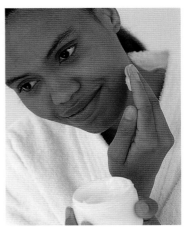

▲ APPLYING OIL-BLENDED SKIN CREAM.

body lotion with ten drops rose essential oil. Pour into a bottle with a tight lid to store. A refreshing, lightly fragranced citrus body lotion can be made in the same way using 175ml/6fl oz unscented body lotion, ten drops grapefruit essential oil and five drops bergamot essential oil; however, do not apply this lotion before going into the sun.

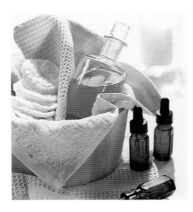

◀ OIL-SCENTED BODY LOTION IS BEST APPLIED AFTER A WARM BATH.

Classic cleansers

Gentle but effective cleansers are easy to make from pure, simple ingredients. Soapwort cleansing liquid is made by placing 15g/½ oz chopped soapwort root (available from herbalists) in a pan with 600ml/1 pint bottled spring water. Bring to the boil and simmer for 15 minutes. Strain the infusion through a paper filter, then stir in 50ml/2fl oz rose water and decant the mixture into a glass bottle. This will keep for one month in the fridge.

Another classic cleanser is almond oil cleanser, which is a traditional mix of beeswax,

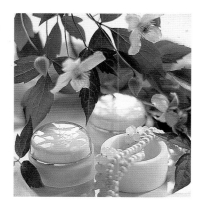

almond oil and rose water. Melt 25g/1oz white beeswax in a double boiler and whisk in 150ml/5fl oz almond oil. In a pan, add 1.5ml/¼ tsp borax (available from chemists) to 60ml/4 tbsp rose water and warm gently to dissolve. Slowly add the rose water mixture to the oils, whisking all the time. Add a few drops of rose essential oil. Continue to whisk until the mixture has a smooth, creamy texture. Pour the cleanser into a container and leave to cool. Replace the lid. To use the cleanser, smooth it on to the skin using a circular movement and remove with damp cotton wool.

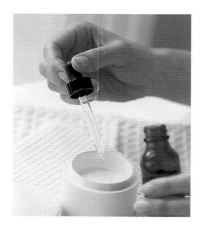

◀ Adding drops of oil to skin cream.

Hand care

Our hands frequently suffer from poor circulation and damage caused from overuse and abuse. Warm hand baths and the application of hand cream relieve poor circulation, soothe the skin and heal any cuts.

HAND BATHS

Circulation to our extremities is affected by tension and stress, among other things. The warmth of the water in a hand bath can help the blood vessels to dilate, which can be helpful in treating tension headaches and migraines, when the blood vessels in the head are frequently engorged with blood. If you regularly suffer from these problems, try a hand bath at the first signs of a headache to drain away the excess stress.

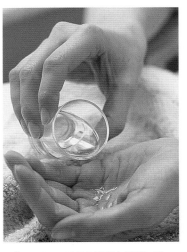

▲ RELAX TIRED HANDS WITH A BLEND OF ROSEMARY AND PINE ESSENTIAL OILS.

▼ A WARM HAND BATH CAN HELP TO RELIEVE POOR CIRCULATION IN THE HANDS.

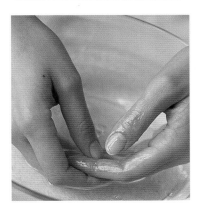

For poor circulation and tense, cold fingers, add two drops lavender and two drops marjoram essential oils to a large bowl two-thirds filled with hot water. Soak your hands in the bowl of water for relief of discomfort.

To relieve over-exertion causing tension and stiffness, try a blend of two drops rosemary and two drops pine in a bowl of hot water.

HAND CREAMS

You can make hand creams by adding suitable essential oils to an unscented cream. Look for a lanolin-rich cream or one that includes cocoa butter as hands benefit from a richer formulation. For a healing cream (see below) blend chamomile, geranium and lemon with unscented hand cream. Store the cream in a plastic bottle.

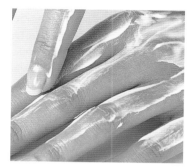

▲ YOU SHOULD ALWAYS TRY TO REMEMBER TO MOISTURIZE YOUR HANDS AT LEAST TWICE A DAY.

PREPARING A HEALING HAND CREAM

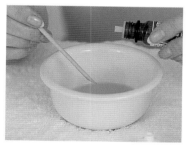

1 Blend ten drops chamomile with five drops geranium and lemon.

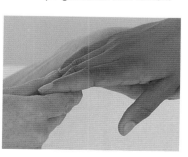

2 Blend the oils with 120ml/4fl oz unscented hand cream.

3 Spread the hand cream over the hands and rub it in thoroughly. The cream is healing because the chamomile oil soothes rough skin, the geranium oil helps heal cuts and the lemon oil softens the skin.

Foot care

Feet often suffer from neglect. We take them for granted, and seldom care for them the way we do the rest of the body. Warming foot baths and soothing foot creams are two ways of relieving neglected feet.

FOOT BATHS

Just as hands can be treated with a warm hand bath, feet can also benefit from a foot bath to which has been added three or four drops of essential oil. The warmth of the water helps circulation to improve and soothes aches and pains.

Peppermint essential oil is cooling, counteracts tiredness and is the ideal oil for using in a refreshing foot bath. For hot, aching feet, add two drops peppermint and two drops lemon oil to a large bowl two-thirds filled with hot water. Soak your feet in the water for instant relief.

If you suffer from poor circulation in your toes, add two drops lavender and two drops marjoram oil to a bowl of hot water. Soak your feet until warmed through.

▼ RELAX WITH A WARM FOOT BATH.

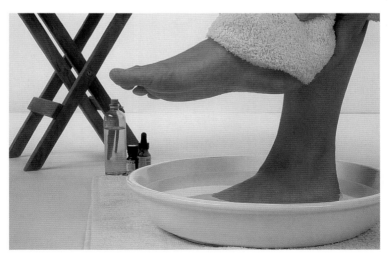

FOOT CREAMS

You can easily make your own
foot cream by adding suitable
essential oils to an unscented
cream. Tea tree is one of the best
essential oils to incorporate in
a foot cream. It has healing,
antiseptic properties as well as a
fungicidal action, which will
protect the feet from the various
foot complaints that can be
picked up at the pool or gym.

To prepare tea tree foot cream,
blend 15 drops tea tree essential
oil thoroughly into 120ml/4fl oz
unscented lanolin-rich cream
(or one that includes cocoa butter).
Pour the blended cream into a
plastic storage bottle using a

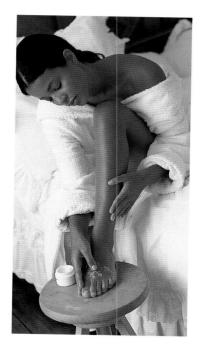

funnel. Although most creams and
lotions are best stored in glass or
ceramic containers, it is more
practical to keep the foot cream in
a pump-action plastic bottle.

To use the foot cream, simply
press the plunger to release
a small amount of cream on
to your hands, and rub all over
your feet to soothe and heal.
Apply as often as required.

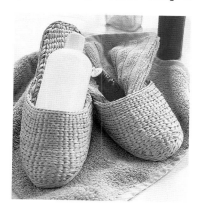

◀ SET ASIDE TIME TO PAMPER YOUR FEET.

Bathing

Imagine soaking in a hot bath, enveloped in a delicious scent of exotic flowers, feeling all the day's tensions drop away . . . well, it can be a reality with aromatherapy. The scented essential oils immediately soothe and relax.

Essential oils make a luxurious addition to the bath, whether they are chosen to aid recovery from a particular illness, to lift the spirits, or to promote relaxation after a stressful day. The essential oils that are recommended for the bath affect the body as they are

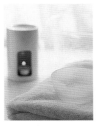

▶ Use essential oil burners to add therapeutic scents to your rooms.

inhaled in the steam, but some will also cling to the skin and penetrate through skin pores that have opened in the warm atmosphere. In order to add the oils to the bath safely it is important to dilute them. There are a variety of ways to do this, the most common of which is to use a vegetable oil – any one of the carrier oils used for massage will be suitable. For those who do not need or like an oily bath, a commercial dispersing agent (available from health food shops), some ordinary dairy cream, or full-fat milk can be used instead. These non-slip carriers are especially important in baths for the elderly and young children.

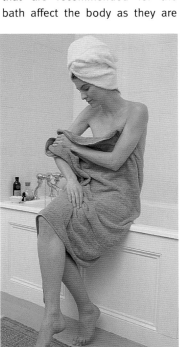

◀ Gently pat your skin dry after a bath.

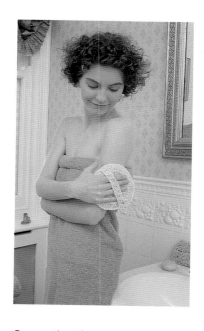

◀ RUBBING THE BODY WITH A LOOFAH INCREASES THE EFFECTIVENESS OF AN AROMATHERAPY BATH.

ylang ylang essential oils to add to your bath. For tired, tense and aching muscles, try soaking in a bath to which you have added three drops marjoram and two drops chamomile essential oils.

Add the blend to the water just before the bath has filled to the desired depth, pouring it in slowly under the hot water tap so that the oil is dispersed through the air and the water. After the bath, gently pat the skin dry with a soft towel. Avoid a vigorous rub-down.

Preparation for an aromatherapy bath should include the removal of dead skin cells. Use a massage mitt or a thoroughly dampened loofah, and rub it firmly but gently over the whole body.

SUGGESTED OIL BLENDS

For a refreshing, uplifting bath in the mornings try a blend of three drops bergamot and two drops geranium essential oils.

To relax and unwind after a long day, make a blend of three drops lavender and two drops

▼ CANDLES CREATE A SENSUAL ATMOSPHERE.

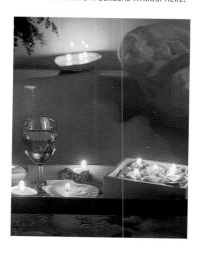

De-stressers

Stress, or rather our inability to cope with an excess amount of it, is one of the biggest health problems today. Regardless of how we react to stress, we can all benefit from the wonderfully balancing effects of aromatic oils.

Our bodies are geared to cope with a stressful situation by producing various hormones that trigger off a series of physiological actions in the body; these are known as the "fight or flight" syndrome, and serve to place the body in a state of alert in a potentially dangerous situation. Extra blood is shunted to the muscles, and the heart rate speeds up while the digestion slows down. These responses are appropriate when we are faced with a physical threat, but can be triggered by quite different kinds of stress and place a strain on our bodies without fulfilling any useful need. In order to help reduce the impact of stress on the whole system, it is necessary to find ways both to avoid getting over-stressed in the first instance and to let go of the changes that occur internally under stress. Aromatherapy can help in each case, the oils helping to keep you calm under pressure and releasing inner tensions following stress, especially in massage. To prevent undue stress, you can try simply inhaling your favourite essential oil at regular intervals throughout the day.

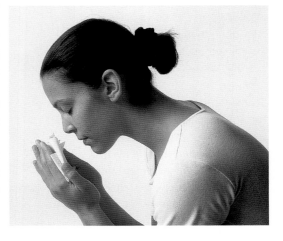

▶ INHALE ESSENTIAL OIL TO RELEASE TENSION.

If possible, use one of the following blends of essential oil in a base oil, and get your partner to massage you, for the perfect antidote to life's stresses. For aiding relaxation, use three drops lavender, three drops geranium and three drops marjoram oils. For calming and soothing, as well as giving a gentle uplift, use four drops rose and three drops jasmine oils. For a more definitely uplifting and energizing effect, try three drops clary sage and four drops bergamot essential oils.

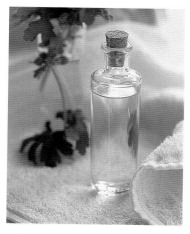

▲ GERANIUM OIL COMBINED WITH LAVENDER AND MARJORAM OILS AIDS RELAXATION.

STRESS-RELIEVING MASSAGE

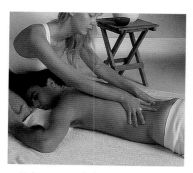

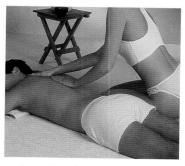

1 Using one of the recommended blends of essential oils, slowly and gently massage the oil into your partner's skin, moving your hands down each side of the spine.

2 For relaxation, use one hand after the other to stroke down the back in a steady rhythm. Continue stroking for several minutes to allow the tension to drain away.

Properties of essential oils

This chart provides a ready reference to those essential oils that are suitable for use in the home, together with some of the more common complaints and disorders they may be used to treat.

	ACHE	ARTHRITIS	ATHLETE'S FOOT	BAD BREATH	BOILS, BLISTERS	BRITTLE NAILS	BROKEN VEINS	BRONCHITIS,	CHEST INFECTIONS	BRUISES	BURNS	CHILBLAINS	COLD SORES	CYSTITIS, URINARY	INFECTIONS	DANDRUFF	DERMATITIS	EARACHE	ECZEMA	
BENZOIN		•							•				•		•					
BERGAMOT	•		•						•			•	•		•			•		
BLACK PEPPER		•																		
CEDARWOOD	•	•							•						•					
CHAMOMILE	•	•			•					•	•	•			•	•		•		
CLARY SAGE	•															•				
CYPRESS									•						•					
EUCALYPTUS		•							•						•					
FENNEL									•											
FRANKINCENSE									•						•					
GERANIUM	•									•	•	•			•	•			•	
GINGER		•																		
GRAPEFRUIT	•																			
JASMINE																				
JUNIPER	•	•													•		•		•	
LAVENDER										•	•							•		
LEMON	•	•			•	•			•	•		•	•							
MANDARIN	•																			
MARJORAM		•							•	•		•								
NEROLI							•		•											
NUTMEG		•																		
ORANGE									•											
PALMAROSA	•														•		•			
PEPPERMINT	•			•					•								•			
ROSE							•											•		
ROSEMARY	•								•							•	•	•		
ROSEWOOD	•																•			
SANDALWOOD	•								•						•				•	
TEA TREE	•		•						•		•		•		•	•		•		
YLANG YLANG																				

FLU	HEAVY PERIODS	HICCUPS	INSECT BITES	IRREGULAR PERIODS	LACK OF PERIODS	MENOPAUSE	MOUTH ULCERS	NEURALGIA	NOSE BLEEDS	PALPITATIONS	PERIOD PAIN	PILES (HAEMORRHOIDS)	PMS	RASHES, ALLERGIES	RHEUMATISM	SCARS	SKIN ULCERS	SORE THROATS	SPOTS	SPRAINS, STRAINS	THRUSH	WARTS, VERRUCAS	WOUNDS, CUTS, SORES
•							•							•	•			•					•
•			•															•	•		•		•
•								•							•								
															•								
		•		•			•				•		•	•	•					•	•		
					•						•		•					•					
•	•						•				•	•			•								
•			•																				
		•			•	•	•						•		•								
•	•										•			•	•	•	•	•			•		•
				•		•											•	•					•
•			•		•										•			•		•			
•													•										
				•							•		•		•			•		•			
•					•						•	•			•								•
•			•		•						•				•								•
•			•				•		•			•		•	•			•	•		•	•	•
	•																		•				
					•						•		•		•						•		
•						•	•			•			•										
															•								
•							•																
											•				•						•		•
•											•												
			•								•	•			•								
•			•								•	•			•								
																		•					•
																		•					•
•			•				•								•			•	•		•	•	•
									•														

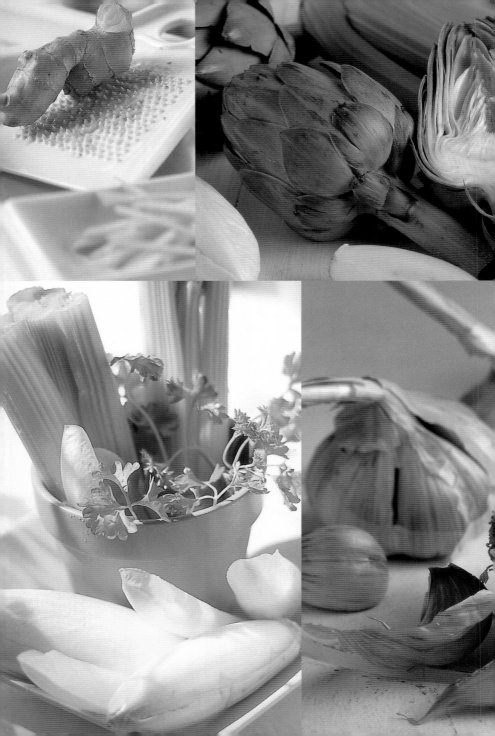

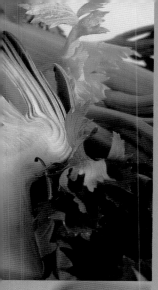

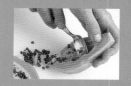

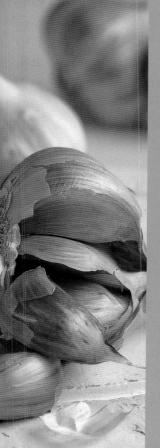

HEALING WITH
FOOD

Eating foods that promote good health makes sense, and is surprisingly simple. This section helps you to make sensible dietary choices, like eating moderate amounts of carbohydrates, sufficient protein, lots of fruits and vegetables, and limiting the amount of salt, sugar and fat you consume on a daily basis.

Aided by the following profiles on fruits, vegetables, pulses, nuts and cereals, you will be able to select the best sources of fibre, protein, vitamins, minerals and antioxidants, and to store and prepare foods to maximize their nutritional value. And what better way to eat for good health than to try out exciting new recipes? The suggestions on the following pages make for simple, easy-to-prepare and delicious fare!

Eating for good health

What we eat has a profound effect on our health and well-being. In a world that is becoming increasingly polluted, and where individuals are subject to high levels of stress, it is easy for our bodies to become out of kilter.

There is ample evidence of a link between poor diet and serious medical conditions like coronary heart disease, cancer and strokes, but it is not just these major health problems that we should be concerned about. A condition does not have to be life threatening to have a huge impact on the way we feel.

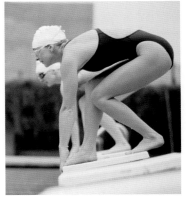

▲ INCORPORATING EXERCISE INTO YOUR DAILY ROUTINE WILL HELP YOUR BODY TO BURN UP EXCESS FAT, IMPROVING BODY TONE.

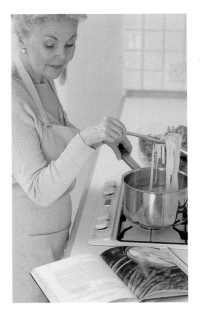

Whatever ails us, whether it is the occasional headache or sore throat, an ongoing condition like diabetes or a digestive problem that causes embarrassment and distress, specific foods can have a positive impact when eaten as part of a sensible, well-balanced diet.

◀ TRYING OUT NEW, HEALTHY RECIPES IS BOTH REWARDING AND ENJOYABLE.

▶ A LOW-FAT MEDITERRANEAN DIET CONSISTING OF FISH, FRESH VEGETABLES AND FRUIT, OLIVE OIL AND A SMALL AMOUNT OF RED WINE PROMOTES GOOD CIRCULATION.

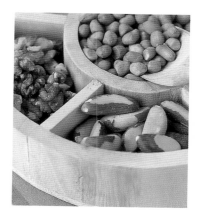
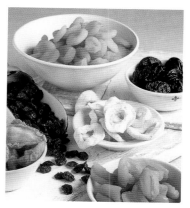

▲ Left and right: Choose healthy snacks that nurture your body, instead of reaching for snacks with empty calories.

Making relatively small changes to our diet, such as eating fruit for a mid-morning snack, can improve matters considerably.

It is important to seek professional advice from a doctor, nutritionist, dietician or state-registered medical specialist before making major changes to your diet, particularly if you are taking any kind of medication.

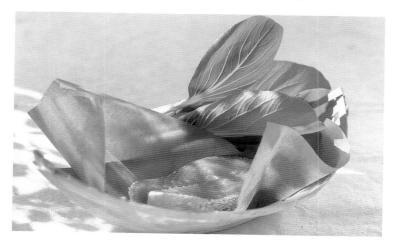

Superfoods

Some foods are such a rich source of concentrated nutrients that they have earned themselves the title "superfoods". Some, such as tofu, are old favourites; others, such as quinoa, have only recently received widespread acclaim.

To understand why these foods are so special, it is useful to look at recent scientific research. One of the most exciting discoveries has been the presence in plants of thousands of different chemical compounds. Each of these compounds – known collectively as phytochemicals – has its own function, and it is believed that some of them may play a crucial role in preventing diseases like cancer, heart disease, arthritis and hypertension. To get the best benefit from phytochemicals, eat at least five different types of fruit and vegetables daily, plus wholegrains, pulses, nuts and seeds.

▼ BUY VEGETABLES IN SMALL QUANTITIES AND EAT THEM AT THEIR FRESHEST.

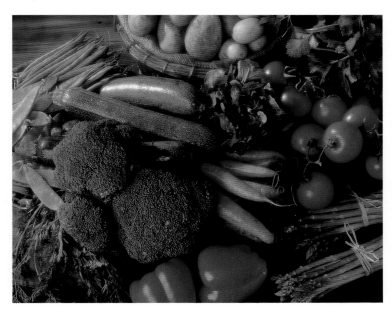

A number of phyto-chemicals also have antioxidant proper-ties. Antioxidants are vital for limiting damage to body cells by unstable molecules known as free radicals. The main antioxidant nutri-ents are vitamins A, C and E, and the minerals zinc and selenium.

When we chew, our bodies produce enzymes. These are protein molecules and are responsible for every aspect of metabolism or the energy we produce. Producing plenty of enzymes improves digestion, detox-ification and immunity, and helps to slow down the aging process.

◀ QUINOA (LEFT) IS A COMPLETE PROTEIN AND HAS A MILD, SLIGHTLY BITTER TASTE AND FIRM TEXTURE. COOK IT IN THE SAME WAY AS RICE. MILLET (BELOW) IS A HIGHLY NUTRITIOUS GLUTEN-FREE GRAIN.

Many of the superfoods highlighted in the pages that follow are excellent sources of enzymes and phytochemicals. Others are included because they contribute valuable minerals, vitamins or omega-3 fatty acids, which are important allies in reducing the risk of heart disease.

▼ STRAWBERRIES ARE RICH IN B COMPLEX VITAMINS AND VITAMIN C. THEY CONTAIN SIGNIFICANT AMOUNTS OF POTASSIUM, AND HAVE GOOD SKIN-CLEANSING PROPERTIES.

GOOD SOURCES OF ANTIOXIDANTS
- Sweet potatoes
- Carrots
- Watercress
- Broccoli
- Peas
- Citrus fruit
- Watermelon
- Strawberries
- Nuts and Seeds

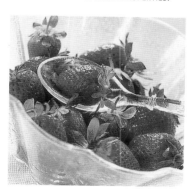

Fruit

What easier way to help yourself to good health than to eat plenty of fruit? There are so many different varieties, with glowing colours and delectable flavours, that eating the recommended portions daily is pure pleasure.

For maximum nutrition, eat fruit that is ripe and freshly picked. Choose lots of different varieties, as each offers many different benefits.

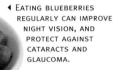

◄ EATING BLUEBERRIES REGULARLY CAN IMPROVE NIGHT VISION, AND PROTECT AGAINST CATARACTS AND GLAUCOMA.

Fruit provides soluble fibre in the form of pectin, which aids digestion and helps to cleanse the liver. All fruits contain generous quantities of antioxidant vitamins C and E, phyto-chemicals and beta-carotene, which the body converts to vitamin A. They help to prevent the furring up of the arteries that leads to atherosclerosis and, in addition, support the

▼ SUMMER PRODUCES AN ABUNDANT CROP OF DELICIOUS SOFT FRUITS.

▼ FRUIT IS THE ULTIMATE CONVENIENCE FOOD, AND AN EXCELLENT SOURCE OF FIBRE.

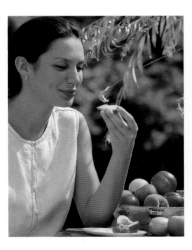

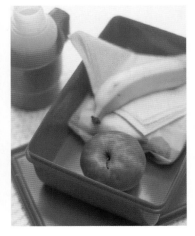

▶ Blackcurrants are usually served
cooked and have a tart flavour.

body's defence system. The antioxidants in fruit may also ease the discomfort of arthritis sufferers by mopping up free radicals and helping to promote the growth of new cartilage. Mangoes, apricots, apples and bananas are particularly useful in this regard.

Apples contain the flavonoid quercetin, which may reduce the risk of heart attacks and strokes.

Bananas are a good source of fibre, vitamins and minerals, especially potassium, which is important for nerve, cell and muscle function, and can help to relieve high blood pressure. Bananas have a high starch content so provide sustained energy. They are a source of tryptophan, an amino acid that lifts the spirits and aids sleep. Ripe bananas strengthen the stomach lining against acid and ulcers.

Blackcurrants are high in antioxidants, vitamins C and E, and carotenes. They contain fibre, and the minerals calcium, iron and

▼ Fresh fruit salad is a healthy and
nutritious dessert.

HOW MUCH IS A PORTION?

Nutritionists recommend eating five portions of fruit and vegetables a day, but what is a portion?
• One medium apple, banana or orange
• A wine glass of any fresh fruit juice
• One large slice of any type of melon or pineapple
• Two plums or kiwi fruit
• About 115g/4oz/1 cup berries

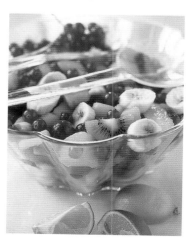

magnesium. Blackcurrants are useful for treating stomach upsets.

Citrus fruits, melons and kiwi fruit are rich in vitamin C, offering relief to asthmatics and people suffering from a wide range of respiratory problems. The membranes of citrus fruit contain pectin, which helps to reduce cholesterol, and also bioflavonoids, which have powerful antioxidant properties.

Figs have laxative qualities and are a good source of calcium.

Gooseberries are rich in vitamin C and also contain betacarotene, potassium and fibre.

Mangoes and apricots contain betacarotene, which may help to prevent inflammation of the lungs and airways. Mangoes are reputed to cleanse the blood, while apricots are a valuable source of vitamin A.

Papaya or pawpaw contains an enzyme called papain, which aids digestion. This fruit contains vitamin C, promoting healthy skin, hair and nails.

Raspberries are a rich source of vitamin C. Eat them to alleviate menstrual cramps. They cleanse the body and remove harmful toxins.

Strawberries cleanse the skin. They are rich in B complex vitamins and vitamin C.

Tomatoes ripened on the vine have higher levels of vitamin C than those picked when green. They contain vitamin E, betacarotene, magnesium, calcium and phosphorus. They aid digestion, reduce blood pressure and lower the risk of developing asthma. Tomatoes contain lycopene, which is believed to prevent some forms of cancer.

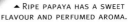

▲ RIPE PAPAYA HAS A SWEET FLAVOUR AND PERFUMED AROMA.

BAKED APPLES

For a nutritious dessert, try these tasty baked apples stuffed with dried fruit and nuts.

INGREDIENTS

4 cooking apples
115g/4oz/²⁄₃ cup mixed dried fruit and nuts
20ml/4 tsp soft dark brown sugar
butter

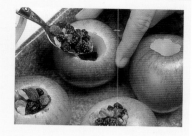

1 Preheat the oven to 180°C/350°F/Gas 4. Remove the core from the apples, score them round their middles, then place them in a baking dish.

2 Mix the fruit, nuts and sugar together and fill the centre of each apple. Pour a little water around the apples and top each with a knob (pat) of butter.

3 Bake for 40–60 minutes, until soft and golden. Serve hot, with low-fat yogurt. Serves 4.

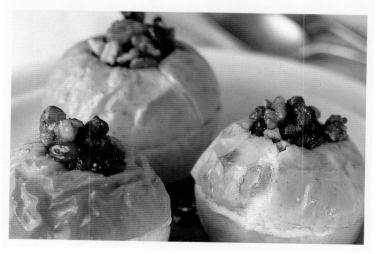

Vegetables

One of the easiest ways of boosting your intake of fibre, vitamins and minerals is to eat plenty of vegetables. Buy organic produce where possible, and make sure it is fresh by purchasing produce from a store with a fast turnover.

Box schemes, run by independent suppliers or co-operatives, are an excellent idea. You state how much you want to spend and how often you would like a delivery, and boxes of beautiful produce arrive on your doorstep regularly. You may be able to specify what they contain, but it can be more fun to have a little of whatever is being harvested. That way you get to try some unfamiliar vegetables.

Like fruit, all vegetables contain phytochemicals, the plant compounds that stimulate the body's enzyme defences against carcinogens (the substances that cause cancer). The best sources are broccoli, cabbages, kohlrabi, radishes, cauliflower, Brussels sprouts, watercress, turnips, kale, pak choi (bok choy), mustard greens, spring

▼ CRUCIFEROUS VEGETABLES ARE PACKED WITH PHYTOCHEMICALS.

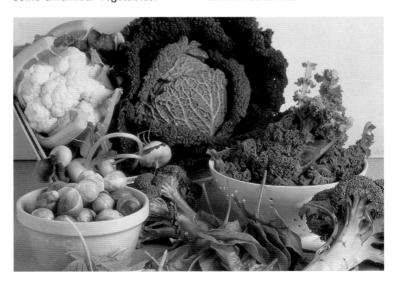

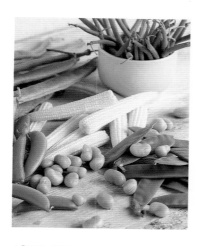

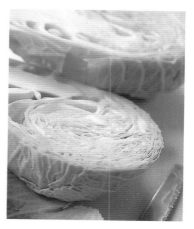

▲ BEANS, PEAS AND CORN CAN BE ENJOYED ALL YEAR ROUND, FRESH OR FROZEN.

▲ CABBAGE IS BEST EATEN RAW. IT IS A VALUABLE SOURCE OF VITAMINS C AND E.

greens (collards), chard and swede (rutabaga). Vegetables are also a good source of antioxidants.

Artichokes are good liver cleansers. A source of vitamins A and C, fibre, iron, calcium and potassium, they are used in natural medicine to treat high blood pressure.

Asparagus has anti-inflammatory properties and helps to soothe painful joints.

Beetroot (beet), when eaten raw, helps to cleanse the liver and is good for detoxifying the skin.

Cabbage has antiviral and antibacterial qualities and is particularly useful raw or juiced. It is thought to speed up the metabolism of oestrogen in women and may protect against breast cancer or cancer of the womb.

Carrots and sweet potatoes are rich in betacarotene, which may help to prevent inflammation of the lungs and airways, and may also ease painful conditions of the joints, such as arthritis.

Chillies are very high in vitamin C. They can help to thin mucus and relieve congested airways, and also stimulate the circulation.

Fennel aids digestion, is a diuretic and has a calming and toning effect on the stomach.

Garlic has been found to lower blood cholesterol levels, reduce

vegetables **191**

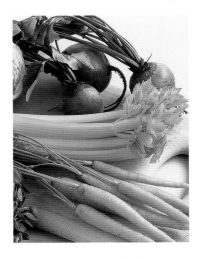

▲ Carrots and beetroot (beet) help the liver to detoxify the body.

possibly prevent asthma attacks. Onions also contain quercetin, an anti-inflammatory that can ease painful joints.

Peas and beans are a good source of protein and fibre. They also contain vitamin C, iron, thiamine, folate, phosphorous and potassium.

Peppers contain plenty of vitamin C, as well as betacarotene, some B complex vitamins, calcium, phosphorous and iron.

Salad leaves are largely composed of water, but are worth eating for

blood pressure and help to prevent the formation of blood clots. An antiviral and antibacterial allium, garlic strengthens the immune system. It is a nasal decongestant. It is best eaten raw, but cooking does not radically decrease its decongestant properties.

Green vegetables that are rich in folic acid may help to lower the risk of heart disease by reducing levels of the amino acid, homocysteine. (High levels are linked to increased risk of coronary heart disease.)

Onions have long been considered a folk cure for respiratory problems. They help clear the airways and

▶ Fennel has a mild aniseed flavour.

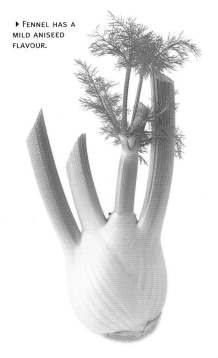

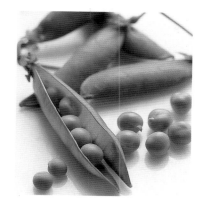

the vitamins and minerals they contribute to the diet. Choose the outer, darker leaves of lettuces, as they are more nutritious than the pale leaves in the centre.

▲ PEAS PICKED AND EATEN FRESH FROM THE POD HAVE A DELICIOUS SWEET TASTE.

▼ ASPARAGUS HAS MILD DIURETIC AND LAXATIVE PROPERTIES.

Spinach is a rich source of cancer-fighting antioxidants, fibre and vitamins C and B6. It also contains calcium, potassium, folate, thiamine, zinc and four times more betacarotene than broccoli.

▼ GARLIC IMPARTS A STRONGER FLAVOUR INTO COOKING WHEN USED CRUSHED.

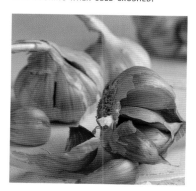

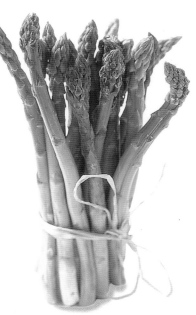

Sprouted grains, seeds and pulses

Sprouted seeds are powerhouses of nutrition. Once the seed, pulse or grain germinates, the nutritional value rockets – by as much as 30 per cent in the case of B vitamins, and 60 per cent for vitamin C.

Sprouts supply plenty of protein, vitamin E, potassium and phosphorus. You can buy sprouts from supermarkets, but they'll be fresher – and cost less – if you grow them. Children love watching them germinate, they taste good in fresh and cooked dishes, and they are very easy to digest.

Many seeds, pulses (legumes) and grains can be sprouted successfully. Here are some of the best.

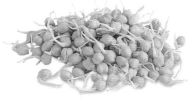

▲ CHICKPEA SPROUTS

Chickpea sprouts are deliciously nutty, but take longer to sprout than small beans. They must be rinsed four times a day.

▼ LENTIL SPROUTS

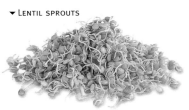

Lentil sprouts are slightly spicy and peppery. Use whole (not split) red,

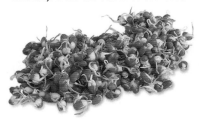

▲ ADUKI BEANSPROUTS

Aduki beansprouts are said to be good for cleansing the system. These fine, feathery sprouts have a sweet, nutty flavour.
Alfalfa sprouts are wispy little sprouts with a nutty, mild flavour. They are best eaten raw.

▼ ALFALFA SPROUTS

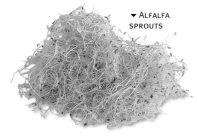

green and brown lentils. They are best eaten when young.

▼ MUNG BEANSPROUTS

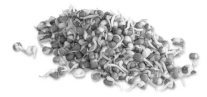

Mung beansprouts are large, with a delicate flavour and crunchy texture. They are great in salads.

▼ WHEAT BERRY SPROUTS

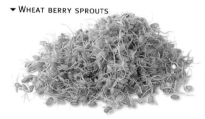

Wheat berry sprouts are sweet and crunchy. They taste great in breads.

STORING SPROUTS
Use sprouts as soon as possible after growing or buying. If you must store them, put them in a plastic bag or sealed tub in the refrigerator. They will keep for 2–3 days. Wash and drain bought sprouts before using them.

SPROUTING

There's nothing simpler than sprouting seeds. It's the fastest way to grow your own organic produce. Most seeds are ready to eat in 3–4 days.

1 Rinse 45ml/3 tbsp seeds, pulses (legumes) or grains, drain and place in a clean jar. Fill with lukewarm water, cover with muslin and fasten securely. Leave in a warm place overnight.

2 Pour off the water, leaving the muslin in place. Refill with water, shake gently, then drain as before. Leave the jar in a warm place, away from direct sunlight.

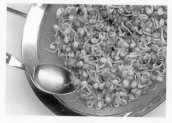

3 Rinse and drain three times a day until they have grown to the desired size. Remove from the jar, rinse, drain and discard any that haven't germinated.

Sea vegetables

For centuries, Asian cooks have known about the health benefits of sea vegetables such as arame, laver and kombu, but the Western world is just waking up to the potential of including these valuable superfoods in the diet.

Sea vegetables are an excellent source of betacarotene and contain some of the B complex vitamins. They are rich in minerals. Calcium, magnesium, potassium, phosphorus and iron are all present, and are credited with boosting the immune system, reducing stress and helping the metabolism to function efficiently. Eating sea vegetables regularly can improve the hair and skin, and the iodine they contribute improves thyroid function and prevents goitre.

Sea vegetables can be used in many different ways. Try toasting them and crumbling them into stir-fries or salads, or add them to soups and casseroles.

Arame is sold as thin, wiry strips. It is mild and slightly sweet.

Dulse is a purple-red sea vegetable which is chewy and tastes spicy. It is rich in potassium, iodine, phosphorous, iron and manganese.

◀ ARAME

Kombu is very versatile, and forms part of the Japanese stock, dashi. It has a strong flavour and is a rich source of iodine.

Laver is a rich source of minerals and vitamins. Cans of laver purée are available from health food stores. Spread it on hot toast.

Nori is a delicately flavoured seaweed that is processed into thin sheets, to be used as wraps. Toast it under a grill (broiler) before use.

Wakame is a versatile sea vegetable, rich in calcium and vitamins B and C. It can also be toasted and crumbled over food.

▼ DULSE

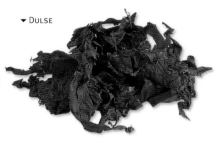

SIMPLE SALMON SUSHI

Sushi is a healthy snack. The rice contributes complex carbohydrate, the fish is a good source of protein and omega-3 fatty acids, and the nori wrapper is a source of iodine.

INGREDIENTS

25ml/1½ tbsp granulated sugar
5ml/1 tsp sea salt
30ml/2 tbsp Japanese rice
  vinegar
250g/9oz/1¼ cups sushi rice
3 sheets yaki nori (toasted
  nori)
175g/6oz very fresh salmon
  fillet, cut into fingers

1 Mix the sugar and salt in a bowl. Add the vinegar and stir until dissolved.

2 Cook the rice according to the instructions on the packet. Drain, add the vinegar mixture and stir well, fanning the rice constantly. Cover with a damp cloth. Cool.

3 Cut the yaki nori in half lengthways and place a half-sheet, shiny side down, on a bamboo mat.

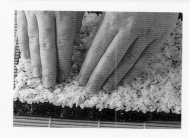

4 Spread with a layer of vinegared rice, leaving a 1cm/½in clear edge at top and bottom. Arrange fingers of salmon across the centre.

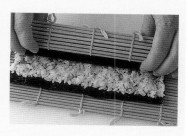

5 Roll up the yaki nori into a cigar. Wrap in clear film and chill.

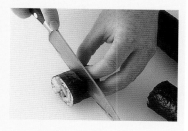

6 Cut into 24 slices.

Cereal grains

The seeds of cereal grasses, grains are packed with concentrated goodness and are an important source of complex carbohydrates, protein, vitamins and minerals. Grains are inexpensive and versatile.

Wheat, rice, oats and barley have always been an important part of the diet, but it is some of the less well-known grains that are currently causing excitement. Two of these are quinoa and millet. Both have been cultivated for centuries, but it is only comparatively recently that the full extent of their nutritional value has been realized.

Millet is highly nutritious. Low in fat, it is easily digested. The grains are a good source of iron, zinc, calcium, manganese and B vitamins.

Oats have been found to lower blood pressure. They provide insoluble fibre, which can reduce blood cholesterol levels when part of a low-fat diet. Oats are a source of vitamin E, an anti-inflammatory.

Quinoa is the only grain that is a complete protein, possessing all eight essential amino acids. Low in saturated fats and high in fibre, it is an excellent source of calcium, potassium, zinc, iron, magnesium and B vitamins. It is cooked like rice, but the grains swell to four times their original size. As the grain cooks, the germ that surrounds it forms a spiral that resembles a bean sprout. This stays firm and crunchy, providing a tasty contrast to the soft, creamy grain. Use quinoa in pilaffs, bakes, stuffings and as a breakfast cereal. It is also available in flakes and as flour.

◀ CLOCKWISE FROM TOP: ROLLED OATS, OATMEAL, WHOLE OATS AND OATBRAN.

◄ BROWN AND WHITE RICE

Wheat is a nutritious grain, but not everyone can tolerate it. It is best eaten unprocessed, as wholewheat. It is a very good source of dietary fibre, most of which is in the bran. It also contains B vitamins, vitamin E, iron, selenium and zinc. Wholegrains are a source of phytoestrogens, which may also help to protect against breast cancer.

Rice is a good source of fibre, vitamins and minerals. Eat brown rice where possible, as it retains the husk, bran and germ in which most of the nutrients reside.

RECIPE SUGGESTION

TABBOULEH

A quick and easy way to boost your dietary fibre intake.

INGREDIENTS

175g/6oz/1 cup bulgur wheat
*30ml/2 tbsp each chopped fresh
  mint and parsley*
6 spring onions (scallions), sliced
½ cucumber, diced
60ml/4 tbsp extra virgin olive oil
juice of 1 large lemon
salt and ground black pepper

1 Place the bulgur wheat in a bowl. Pour on boiling water to cover. Leave to stand for 30 minutes, so that the grains swell.

2 Drain well, removing as much water as possible. Tip the wheat into a bowl.

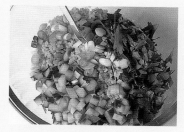

3 Add all the remaining ingredients and toss well. Chill for 30 minutes to allow the flavours to mingle. Serve as a salad, or as a filling for warm wheat tortillas, with guacamole. Serves 4–6.

Pulses

Low in fat and high in complex carbohydrates, vitamins and minerals, pulses are economical, easy to cook and good to eat. They are a valuable source of protein and good for diabetics, as they help to control sugar levels.

LENTILS AND DRIED PEAS

There are several varieties. All these pulses (legumes) are low in fat and rich in protein. They are a good source of fibre and are reputed to help lower levels of harmful LDL cholesterol.

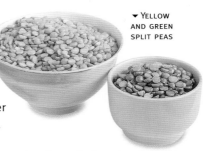

▼ YELLOW AND GREEN SPLIT PEAS

DRIED BEANS

These are packed with protein, soluble and insoluble fibre, iron, potassium, manganese, magnesium, folate and most B vitamins. Soya beans are the superfood here, containing all the amino acids essential for the renewal of cells and tissues. Including dried beans in your diet regularly can lower cholesterol levels, reducing the risk of heart disease and strokes. Beans contain phytoestrogens, which can protect against cancer of the breast, prostate and colon. There are plenty of other varieties too, including aduki beans, black beans, black-eyed beans (peas), borlotti beans, broad (fava) beans, butter (lima) beans, flageolet or cannellini beans, chickpeas, haricot (navy) beans, pinto beans, red kidney beans and ful medames. Canned beans are not as nutritious as dried beans, but contain appreciable amounts of nutrients.

◀ CLOCKWISE FROM LEFT: HARICOT (NAVY) BEANS, KIDNEY BEANS, FLAGEOLET (CANNELLINI) BEANS AND PINTO BEANS.

Split pea mash

This purée makes an excellent alternative to mashed potatoes, and is particularly good with winter pies and nut roasts. Serve warm with pitta bread.

Ingredients

225g/8oz/1 cup yellow split peas, soaked overnight
1 bay leaf
8 sage leaves, roughly chopped
15ml/1 tbsp olive oil
4 shallots, finely chopped
5ml/1 tsp cumin seeds
1 large garlic clove, chopped
50g/2oz/¼ cup butter, softened
salt and ground black pepper

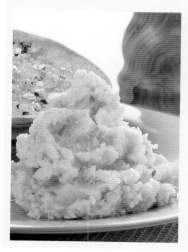

1 Drain the split peas, put them in a pan with cold water to cover and bring to the boil. Skim, add the herbs and simmer for 10 minutes.

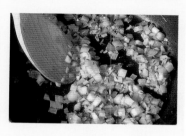

2 Heat the oil and fry the shallots with the cumin seeds and garlic for 3 minutes. Add to the pan and simmer for 30 minutes more. Drain, reserving the cooking water.

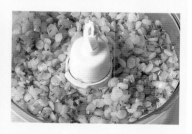

3 Remove the bay leaf, then process the split peas with the butter and enough of the cooking water to form a coarse purée. Season, serve warm with diced tomatoes and olive oil. Serves 4–6.

Protein foods

An essential nutrient, protein is converted by the body into amino acids, which are vital for the growth and repair of body cells. The body manufactures some amino acids, but eight cannot be manufactured.

Eating a good variety of proteins is important because the eight amino acids have to come from our food. The other 12 amino acids can all be synthesised from the food that we eat. Good sources of protein are red meat, poultry, fish, milk, eggs, quinoa, lentils and beans, especially soya beans and their derivatives. Tofu, an excellent source of protein, is a rich source of B vitamins, essential fatty acids,

▼ EAT A VARIETY OF PROTEIN TO ENSURE YOU GET THE MAXIMUM NUTRIENTS.

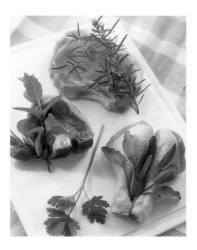

zinc and iron. It contains phyto-estrogens that help to regulate hormone levels, and can lower cholesterol levels if eaten regularly.

Although protein is so important, we do not need to eat vast amounts of it; eating too much protein, especially animal protein, can lead to weight gain and osteoporosis. Far better to balance a moderate amount of animal protein with protein from plant sources, such as tofu, quinoa, rice and pasta. There is also protein in bread and breakfast cereals.

Limit red meat to four 115–175g/ 4–6oz servings a week, and try not to eat more than three eggs. Milk, cheese and yogurt provide protein, calcium and vitamins B12, A and D. Choose low-fat products and consume in moderation.

Eat fish twice a week. Choose oily fish for preference. Herrings, sardines, mackerel, salmon and tuna provide omega-3 fatty acids, which can help to reduce the risk of heart disease.

MOROCCAN SPICED MACKEREL

A spicy marinade is the perfect foil for rich, oily fish.

INGREDIENTS

150ml/¼ pint/⅔ cup sunflower
  oil
15ml/1 tbsp paprika
5–10ml/1–2 tsp chilli powder
10ml/2 tsp ground cumin
10ml/2 tsp ground coriander
2 garlic cloves, crushed
juice of 2 lemons
30ml/2 tbsp chopped fresh mint
30ml/2 tbsp chopped fresh
  coriander (cilantro)
4 mackerel, cleaned
salt and ground black pepper
lemon wedges and mint sprigs,
  to serve

1 Whisk the oil, spices, garlic and lemon juice. Add the herbs.

2 Slash each mackerel in several places, then place in the dish. Turn to coat in the marinade.

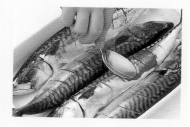

3 Cover with plastic wrap and chill for 3–5 hours. Grill (broil) for 5–7 minutes on each side. Turn once and baste often. Serve with lemon and mint. Serves 4.

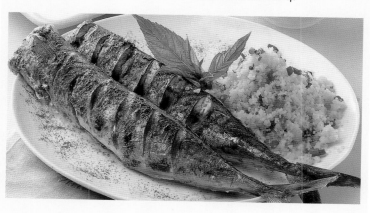

Nuts and seeds

Seeds and nuts make a valuable addition to the diet. Most nuts make delicious snacks, and are tasty sprinkled on salads and desserts. A few almonds, dry-roasted in a frying pan, make a wonderful topping for grilled chicken.

Nuts are an excellent source of B complex vitamins and vitamin E, an antioxidant that has been associated with a lower risk of heart disease, stroke and certain cancers. They are a useful source of protein, but are high in calories, so don't have too many of them.

IN A NUTSHELL

Brazil nuts are high in saturated fat, but cholesterol-free. They are a rich source of selenium, which is a mood enhancer.

Chestnuts contain very little fat and are a good source of potassium.

Peanuts are high in fat, but a good source of potassium. Eat sparingly.

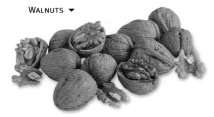

WALNUTS ▼

Pecan nuts have a very high fat content, so eat only occasionally.

Walnuts supply omega-3 fatty acids, which help to keep the heart healthy. Fatty acids thin the blood, which helps to prevent blood clots (DVT) and reduce blood cholesterol levels. They can also reduce inflammation in painful joints. Walnuts are also rich in potassium, magnesium, iron, zinc, copper and selenium.

▼ UNSALTED NUTS OF ANY KIND MAKE A HEALTHY SNACK FOR ANY TIME OF DAY.

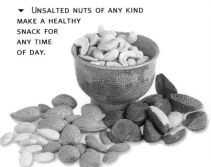

CAUTION
• Always inform guests if you've included nuts in a dish, as some people are highly allergic to them.
• Never eat rancid nuts, as they have been linked to a high incidence of free radicals.

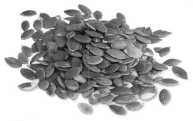

▲ Pumpkin seeds

Seed catalogue

Packed with vitamins and minerals, as well as beneficial oils and protein, seeds make delicious snacks, or can be sprinkled over food to boost the nutritional benefits.

Linseed has abundant levels of omega-3 and omega-6 fatty acids, good for strengthening immunity and easing digestive problems.

Pumpkin seeds are rich in iron and an excellent source of zinc.

Sesame seeds are tiny white or black seeds and are rich in iron.

Sunflower seeds are delicious when dry-roasted. They are a good source of vitamin E and B vitamins and boost flagging energy levels.

▼ Linseeds (left) and hemp seeds

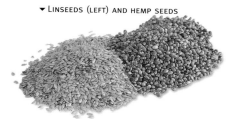

RECIPE SUGGESTION

Salad and roasted seeds
A nutritious light lunch or supper dish.

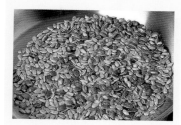

1 Dry-fry 50g/2oz/6 tbsp mixed pumpkin seeds and sunflower seeds in a frying pan, over a high heat, for 3 minutes until golden, tossing frequently to stop them from burning. Set aside to cool slightly.

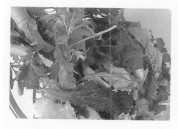

2 Mix about 175g/6oz salad and herb leaves in a bowl. Add the roasted seeds and toss with 30ml/2 tbsp vinaigrette to combine. Serves 4.

Herbs and spices

Herbs and spices are invaluable in the kitchen, not only because they help to make our food taste good without the need for excessive amounts of salt, but also because they are healing foods. Many herbs aid digestion.

Basil helps to relieve stomach cramps, nausea and constipation.

Chillies are an excellent source of vitamin C and a good source of other antioxidants. The spice stimulates the body and is a powerful decongestant.

Cinnamon aids digestion.

Fennel calms the digestive system.

Ginger is an expectorant that helps to fight coughs and colds. It also soothes stomach cramps. Fresh root ginger is an anti-inflammatory, and may help to ease painful joints.

Parsley delivers betacarotene, vitamin B12, ample amounts of vitamin C and a host of minerals, including iron. It aids digestion, can be used as a breath freshener, purifies

◀ ROSEMARY AND SAGE

the blood and supports the liver and the kidneys.

Peppermint is good for digestive problems. A tisane of peppermint and basil can alleviate flatulence.

Rosemary tea is effective against cold symptoms, fatigue and headaches.

Sage is an antiseptic, antibacterial herb. Sage tea eases indigestion and menopausal problems.

Turmeric is an earthy spice that is valued for its antibacterial and anti-fungal properties. Including it in the diet may reduce the risk of certain cancers. It has anti-inflammatory properties, and may ease painful joints.

▼ CHILLIES

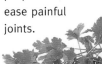

▲ PARSLEY

Foods to avoid

Cut down on foods that are high in saturated fat, including high-fat dairy products, fatty meat and hydrogenated or trans fats found in margarine and processed foods. Drink alcohol in moderation and eat less salt.

If you have respiratory problems, avoid wine, beer, cider, salt, dairy products, wheat, food additives, yeast and red meat. For a weak or compromised immune system, avoid or eat in moderation, dairy products, caffeine, alcohol and processed foods. To ease digestive problems, avoid bran, spicy foods, alcohol and processed foods.

Arthritis sufferers may benefit from cutting down on or eliminating saturated fat and acidic foods, such as citrus fruits. Caffeine, red meat, sugar, alcohol, aubergines (eggplant), tomatoes and potatoes can exacerbate symptoms, so try eliminating these by degrees.

If you are anxious or stressed, avoid or cut down on stimulants, including nicotine, which can deplete the body of valuable nutrients. Alcohol leads to dehydration, and robs the body of vitamins A, C, the B vitamins, magnesium, zinc and essential fatty acids. Tea and coffee inhibit the absorption of iron, magnesium and calcium.

▼ ALCOHOL CAN INHIBIT THE ABSORPTION OF ESSENTIAL VITAMINS AND MINERALS.

▼ CUT DOWN ON THE AMOUNT OF SATURATED FATS THAT YOU EAT.

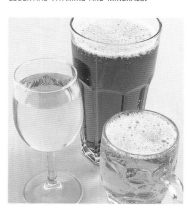

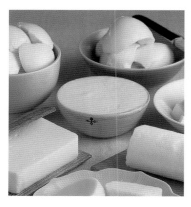

Maximizing nutritional value

To get the most nutritional value from your food, especially fruit and vegetables, it should be as fresh as possible, and any preparation or cooking should ensure that as many nutrients as possible are retained.

• If you grow your own fruit and vegetables, or buy from a farm where the produce is picked or pulled as needed, freshness is guaranteed. If not, make sure your supplier has a rapid turnover.

• Transport produce home quickly. Remove any plastic wrapping. Store produce in a cool larder or in the refrigerator crisper.

• Avoid buying fresh produce from a supermarket or store that has installed fluorescent lighting over displays, as this can cause a chemical reaction, depleting nutrients in fruit and vegetables.

• Buy organic produce where possible, and do not peel it unless absolutely necessary, since nutrients are concentrated just below the skin. Instead wash produce thoroughly. Although prepared vegetables are convenient, it is not a good idea to peel or slice

▾ BUY LOOSE PRODUCE WHEN YOU CAN: IT IS EASIER TO CHECK THAN PRE-PACKED FOOD.

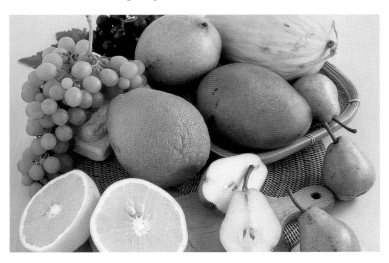

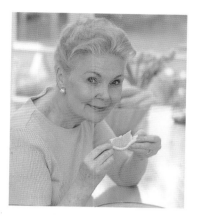

▲ An orange a day supplies an adult
with the daily requirement of vitamin C.

produce until you are ready to use it, as the nutritional value diminishes rapidly after preparation.

• Try to eat most of your vegetables and fruit raw. Otherwise, use a steamer in preference to boiling vegetables since soluble vitamins, such as thiamine and vitamin C and B vitamins leach into the water. If you must boil vegetables, use just a little water, and save the water to use in a soup or sauce.

• Buy nuts and seeds in small quantities. Store them in airtight containers in a cool, dark place. Herbs, spices, pulses (legumes), flours and grains should be kept in the same way. Store oils in a cool, dark place to prevent oxidation.

STORAGE TIPS

Apples Store in a cool place, away from direct sunlight.
Bananas Store bananas at cool room temperature, away from other fruit.
Berries Store in a tub lined with a paper towel, in the refrigerator. Use the same day if possible.
Celery Store in the salad drawer of the refrigerator for 1–2 weeks.
Fennel Keep for 2–3 days in the salad drawer of the refrigerator.
Grapes Store unwashed in the refrigerator for up to 5 days.
Squash Can be kept for several weeks in a cool, dry place. When cut, wrap and store in refrigerator.
Tomatoes Store at room temperature; chilling spoils the taste and texture.

▼ To ripen bananas, store them in a brown paper bag with an already ripe fruit. Keep in a cool, dark place.

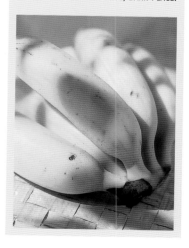

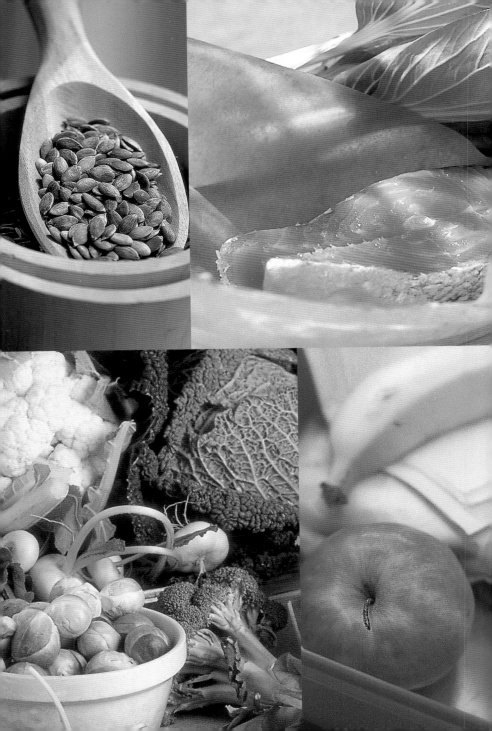

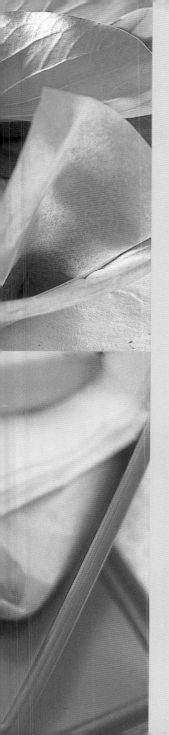

RECIPES FOR
AILMENTS

By thinking more about the food you eat, you
are likely to find that your general well-being
improves: your skin and hair are in top
condition, your body shape finds its natural
proportions, you have lots of energy and are
seldom ill. Even so, there are times when we
all succumb to minor illnesses like coughs and
colds or headaches, or just wake up feeling a
bit tired or down in the dumps.

The good news is that eating specific foods
can be of enormous help in easing all sorts of
everyday ailments, either by helping the
immune system to work more efficiently,
supplying essential nutrients that have been
lacking in the diet, or by helping to restore
balance to a body system under stress.

Easing the symptoms

 If you are not in peak physical condition, the signs often show in the body. Dull, lifeless locks don't necessarily mean merely a bad hair day; they may signal that something more serious is wrong.

Thin or brittle nails, successive mouth ulcers, digestive upsets – all these are indications that all is not as it should be. The problem may be something minor, a health hiccup if you like, but it is also possible that there is a more serious underlying cause. Always see your doctor if symptoms persist or are particularly severe. This book offers some suggestions that may help to prevent certain conditions from developing, and ease those that have, but it is not our intention to suggest that diet can ever be a substitute for professional diagnosis and treatment.

Having said that, there are plenty of practical steps you can take to ease unpleasant symptoms. Imagine sipping a glass of papaya juice next time you have a sore throat. As it goes down, the cool

▼ ALTERNATIVE HEALTH PRACTITIONERS CAN HELP YOU COME TO TERMS WITH AN ILLNESS OR CONDITION BY SUGGESTING DIETARY AND LIFESTYLE CHANGES THAT WILL HELP.

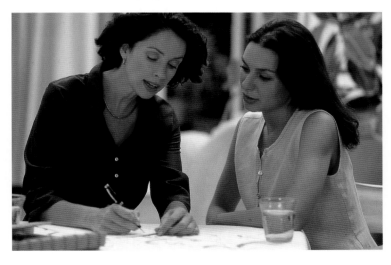

liquid will soothe and comfort, and an enzyme in the fruit will help to alleviate your discomfort. If you have had a bout of diarrhoea, eating live yogurt can help to balance the microflora in the gut. A ripened banana can boost potassium levels and help to bring down high blood pressure.

Nature provides a wonderful natural pharmacy of fruits, vegetables, herbs and spices, which can be of great benefit alongside conventional medical treatment.

▼ EXERCISING HELPS TO KEEP YOU FIT, REDUCES STRESS AND TENSION AND MAKES YOU FEEL BETTER PSYCHOLOGICALLY.

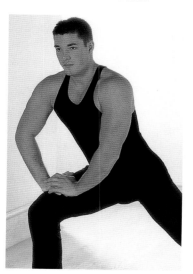

RECIPE SUGGESTION

PAPAYA JUICE SOOTHER
This reviving juice helps the throat, liver and kidneys.
INGREDIENTS
1 papaya
½ cantaloupe melon
90g/3½oz white grapes

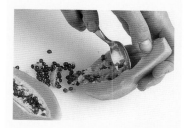

1 Halve and skin the papaya, remove the seeds and cut into rough slices. Cut open the melon and remove the seeds. Slice the flesh away from the skin, then cut into rough chunks.

2 Blend the fruit in a processor.

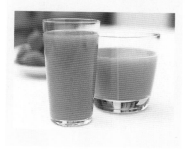

Headaches and migraine

Having a headache is no fun, and when headaches occur regularly, or are particularly severe, they can be worrying as well as unpleasant. If you notice a recurring pattern to your headaches, you need to take action.

If your doctor has ruled out any underlying medical condition, making changes to your diet can make you less prone to headaches, particularly if they are triggered by low blood sugar levels. Erratic eating habits can be a factor, so eat small amounts of healthy food at regular intervals, and don't skip meals.

If you wake up with a thumping headache after a night out, you may be dehydrated so drink plenty of water. Coffee and cola contain caffeine, which affects the blood supply to the brain, and can cause headaches, so drink in moderation.

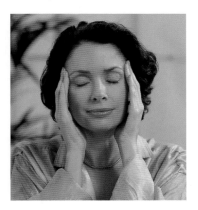

Tension headaches – the kind that make you feel as though your head is trapped in a vice – may be caused by stress. Make sure you are getting your quota of B vitamins by eating wholegrains, dairy products, lean meat, seafood, green vegetables, nuts and seeds. Vitamin C is depleted in times of stress, so eat an orange or a couple of kiwi fruit every day.

MIGRAINE

Some migraine attacks appear to be triggered by a reaction to a specific food, with chocolate, cheese, coffee and citrus fruits the main culprits. Alcohol, especially red wine, may also be implicated, and there are suggestions that stock cubes, processed meats containing nitrates and even pulses (legumes) can be problematical for some sufferers. Food allergies can be a trigger; if you think this may be the case, seek advice.

◀ DON'T IGNORE A HEADACHE, PARTICULARLY IF YOU ARE A REGULAR SUFFERER.

Vital veggie blends

One of the great cure-all super-foods, broccoli is bursting with vitamins A, B and C, and contains almost as much calcium as milk. When eaten raw or juiced, however, its relatively strong flavour does need a bit of toning down by blending with sweeter ingredients. The following restorative fruit-and-vegetable blend, with its dash of citrus tang, is quick and easy to make, and works hard to replenish vitamins and rehydrate the body. It's an ideal cure for many types of headache.

▼ Broccoli is packed with nutrients and blends beautifully with fruit.

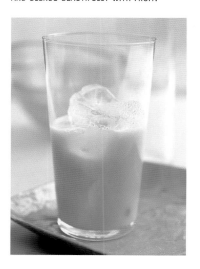

Broccoli booster

The following recipe makes one glass. Juice the florets only and discard the tough stalk.

Ingredients
125g/4¼oz broccoli florets
2 eating apples
15ml/1 tbsp lemon juice
ice cubes

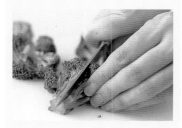

1 Cut the broccoli florets into small pieces and chop the apples.

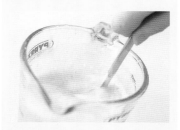

2 Push both through a juicer, stir in the lemon juice, and serve.

Colds and sore throats

Colds are especially common in winter, and characterized by streaming eyes, a sore throat, blocked nose, headaches, aching muscles and a high temperature. Getting plenty of rest and taking care of your health will speed your recovery.

A healthy lifestyle, plenty of exercise and a balanced diet won't stop you getting coughs and colds, but it will help to build up your resistance. You are also likely to recover more rapidly than someone who is below par. If you do succumb, the best advice is to drink plenty of fluids, alternating water with fresh citrus juices. There is some evidence that foods that are rich in zinc can help you fight off a cold. Oysters are the best source, but may not slide down a sore throat all that readily. Try soft scrambled eggs, another source of zinc.

A hot toddy with lemon is an old favoured recipe based on sound nutritional sense. Lemons, like limes, are rich in vitamin C, and have potent antiseptic qualities, making them ideal for combating sore throats and sniffles. Alternatively, try papaya juice, which is great for soothing a sore throat. Reduce dairy produce, which tends to increase mucus production.

If your throat is fine, and you just have a heavy cold, a curry may be just what you need. Include ginger, which is an expectorant, and chilli, a powerful decongestant.

▼ REGARDED AS ONE OF LIFE'S LUXURIES, OYSTERS ARE RICH IN ZINC.

▼ EGGS PROVIDE VITAMINS AND IRON, AND ARE DELICIOUS SCRAMBLED.

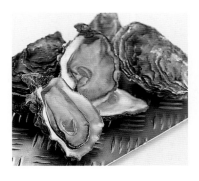

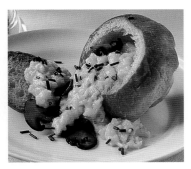

SCAMBLED EGGS IN BRIOCHES

If you do not have any brioches to hand, simply use thick slices of toasted bread. For an indulgent treat when not suffering from a cold, you can also cook the eggs in butter. Serves four.

INGREDIENTS

4 individual brioches
6 eggs, beaten
30ml/2 tbsp chopped fresh
  chives, plus extra to serve
30ml/2 tbsp olive oil
salt and ground black pepper

1 Preheat the oven to 180°C/ 350°F/Gas 4. Slice the tops off the brioches and scoop out the middle. Bake the brioche cases and lids for 5 minutes.

2 Beat the eggs with the chives while heating the olive oil in a pan. Add the egg mixture to the pan and cook, stirring, until semi-solid.

3 Spoon the egg mixture into the brioches, sprinkle with chives, place the lids on the top and serve immediately.

THE BEST HOT TODDY

This irresistible mix of lemon, honey and whisky will help to ease even the most miserable of colds. Makes two glasses.

INGREDIENTS

2 strips of pared lemon rind
4 slices of fresh root ginger
5ml/1 tsp honey
175ml/6fl oz/3/4 cup water
175ml/6fl oz/3/4 cup Scotch
  whisky, Irish whiskey or
  American bourbon

1 Put the lemon rind, ginger, honey and water in a small pan and bring to the boil. Remove from the heat and leave to infuse for 5 minutes.

2 Stir the alcohol into the pan and allow time for it to warm through. Strain before serving.

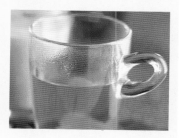

A healthy digestive system

To break down food we need friendly bacteria and digestive enzymes. These are produced by the stomach and small intestine and can get out of balance due to poor diet, stress, antibiotics, food intolerances or toxin overload.

If we suffer these conditions then food remains semi-digested and conditions such as constipation, nausea, flatulence and indigestion can arise. If you are prone to digestive problems, avoid spicy foods, alcohol and processed foods, which can all irritate the gut.

CONSTIPATION

This is a common problem. If there is no underlying medical condition, it may be the result of poor diet, inadequate fluid intake and a

▼ GINGER CAN HELP TO SOOTHE STOMACH CRAMPS. TRY A GINGER AND PEPPERMINT TEA.

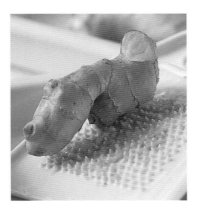

sedentary lifestyle. If you make sure you get enough fibre, drink plenty of water and take some exercise, symptoms can often be alleviated naturally, which is better than resorting to laxatives.

Fresh fruit and vegetables, which are good sources of soluble fibre, stimulate the digestive system, but avoid beans, cabbage and Brussels sprouts, which can cause flatulence and indigestion. Other foods that can boost your fibre levels are brown rice, dried fruit, wholegrain bread and pasta. Bananas are also useful. They are a natural, gentle laxative, and can help to prevent and treat indigestion, and also ulcers.

Eating live natural yogurt can improve the condition of the gut and treat gastro-intestinal disorders. Live yogurt contains active, beneficial bacteria, which balance the intestinal microflora and promote good digestion, boost the immune system and increase resistance to infection.

Soothing smoothie

The following remedy is an easily digested blend of banana, fruit juices and wheatgerm, which will gently soothe a sore or slightly puffy stomach while giving the whole body a boost. Wheatgerm, the most nutritious part of the wheat grain, is packed with B and E vitamins, protein and minerals, while the linseeds contain essential fatty acids that are good for the heart. Be sure to use yogurt with probiotic bacteria to restore balance in the body, although dairy products are best avoided if you are suffering from an inflammation of the gut or diarrhoea, in which case the same amount of non-dairy (soya) yogurt can be substituted.

▼ Banana smoothie is delicious as well as beneficial.

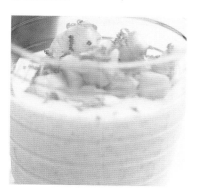

RECIPE SUGGESTION

Classic banana smoothie

This banana body-booster makes one large glass.

Ingredients

30ml/2 tbsp wheatgerm
1 large banana, chopped
130g/4½oz/½ cup live yogurt
15ml/1 tbsp linseeds (flax seeds)
juice of 1 lime
juice of 1 large orange
linseeds and grated lime rind
   to decorate

1 Put the wheatgerm, two-thirds of the banana, the yogurt and linseeds in a blender or food processor. Blend until smooth.

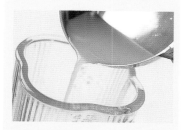

2 Add the lime and orange juice to the yogurt mixture and blend well. Pour into a large glass, top up with mineral water and sprinkle over the lime rind, linseeds and the remaining banana.

Irritable bowel syndrome

It is important to see a doctor if you think you may be suffering from IBS, as similar symptoms may indicate other medical conditions. Symptoms include stomach cramps, bloating, constipation and diarrhoea.

If you have been diagnosed with IBS, there are several steps you can take, such as eating live yogurt, which may make you more comfortable. Have plenty of fruit and vegetables, which contain soluble fibre, but avoid cabbage, lentils and beans. Avoid insoluble fibre, such as wheat bran, particularly in break-fast cereals. Also make sure you drink six glasses of water every day.

Linseed can be helpful. Dissolve 15ml/1 tbsp linseeds in 250ml/8fl oz/1 cup warm water and leave overnight. Next morning, strain into a mug and drink the liquid.

In some people, IBS may be linked to food intolerance. If you suspect this, seek professional advice. An elimination diet may help to pinpoint the problem – a nutritionist should advise you.

TIP
To treat a digestive upset, try grated apple or a glass of apple juice.

▼ HERBAL TEAS AND TISANES, ESPECIALLY CHAMOMILE OR PEPPERMINT, CAN HELP IBS.

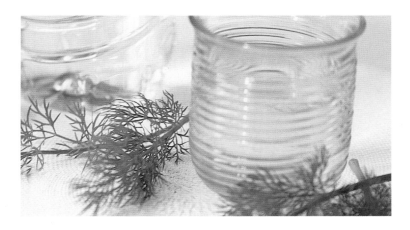

Mouth ulcers

Having a mouth ulcer may not be a major life problem, but it can make you feel pretty miserable as you worry it with your tongue, or try to avoid chewing close to the affected area and biting it with your teeth.

What causes these agonizing little spots is not always clear. They can be the result of an iron deficiency, or failure to take in enough B vitamins, but they might be linked to pre-exam nerves or a similar stressful event. Ill-fitting dentures may be to blame, or a broken tooth. They can also be triggered by a food intolerance.

If you suffer from recurrent clusters of mouth ulcers, it is a good idea to see your doctor, as they may be symptoms of disease.

Take a look at your diet, too. It may be helpful to increase your intake of B vitamins by eating more wholegrains, pulses (legumes), meat and milk. Liver is particularly useful, and will also boost your iron intake, especially if eaten with a source of vitamin C. Liver also contains folate, which is essential for the formation of new body cells, and helps to keep the lining of the mouth healthy. Other sources are pulses, wholegrain cereals and green vegetables.

▼ WHOLEGRAIN CEREALS ARE KNOWN TO HELP PREVENT MOUTH ULCERS.

▼ YOU MAY BE MORE SUSCEPTIBLE TO MOUTH ULCERS IF YOU ARE FEELING LOW.

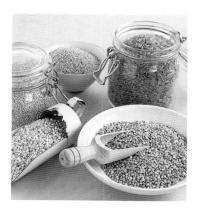

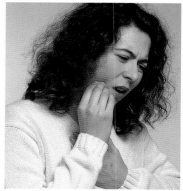

Healthy hair and scalp

Glossy, shiny hair is synonymous with good health, a fact that manufacturers of shampoo capitalize upon. The first step to beautiful hair and a healthy scalp is to eat a well-balanced diet, with plenty of fresh fruit and vegetables.

Aim for a good balance of protein foods, including dairy produce, nuts and pulses (legumes). Your shopping list should include organic artichokes, sweet potatoes, carrots, spinach, broccoli, asparagus and beetroot (beet). Choose apricots, citrus fruits, kiwi fruit, berries and apples. Have plenty of oily fish, and shellfish. Drink six glasses of water a day, and limit sugar.

Dry hair and an itching, flaky scalp may be the result of zinc deficiency. The most efficient way to address this is to swallow an oyster (a single oyster yields 18mg zinc, more than most people consume in a day). Other forms of shellfish are good sources of zinc, too, as are red meat and pumpkin seeds. Essential fatty acids in vegetable oils, nuts and oily fish can also improve the condition of the scalp, while the minerals in sea vegetables, such as kombu and arame, help to make hair lustrous.

Vitamins A and B are important if hair is to be shiny and healthy. Eating liver once a week is a great way of boosting your intake of vitamin A (retinol), provided that you are not pregnant. Fish liver oils are the richest source of retinol, but it can be obtained from eggs and full-cream milk. Also eat carrots, spinach, sweet (bell) peppers, sweet potatoes, peaches and dried apricots on a regular basis. These contain betacarotene, which the body converts to vitamin A.

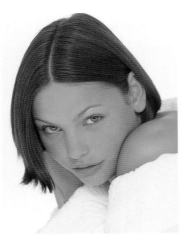

◀ GLOSSY HAIR IS ONE OUTWARD SIGN OF A HEALTHY PERSON.

ARTICHOKES COOKED WITH GARLIC
AND LEMON

This is a very easy way of cooking globe artichokes – the only effort required is in peeling them! Serves four.

INGREDIENTS

4 globe artichokes
juice of 1–2 lemons, plus extra
  to acidulate water
60ml/4 tbsp extra virgin
  olive oil
1 onion, chopped
5–8 garlic cloves, roughly
  chopped or thinly sliced
30ml/2 tbsp chopped fresh
  parsley
120ml/4fl oz/½ cup dry white
  wine
120ml/4fl oz/½ cup vegetable
  stock or water

1 Prepare the artichokes. Pull back the tough leaves until they snap off. Peel the tender part of the stems and cut into bitesize pieces, then put in a bowl of acidulated water. Cut the tops of the artichokes into quarters and scoop out the thistle heart. Add the quarters to the bowl.

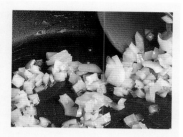

2 Fry the onion and garlic in the oil for 5 minutes until soft. Stir in the parsley, wine, stock, drained artichokes and about half the lemon juice.

3 Bring the mixture to the boil, then cover and simmer for 10–15 minutes until the artichokes are tender. Remove the artichokes and transfer to a serving dish.

4 Boil the cooking liquid until reduced to about half in volume. Pour over the artichokes, drizzle with lemon juice and serve.

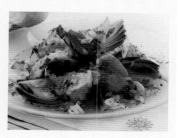

Improving your skin

The skin is the largest organ of the body, and is especially vulnerable to the effects of modern living. The most useful thing you can do to improve the quality of your skin is to drink water; ideally six to eight large glasses every day.

Also of benefit is regular exercise and plenty of fresh air, so a bracing walk in the country is ideal. If you have a specific skin condition, such as eczema or acne, it is important to consult your doctor, but if you merely think your skin is looking a bit lifeless and could do with a lift, you may find the following advice helpful.

Eat fresh vegetables, especially carrots, spinach, broccoli and sweet potatoes, which deliver the antioxidant betacarotene. Citrus fruit, kiwi fruit, berries (especially strawberries), avocados, vegetable oils, wholegrains, nuts, seeds and some types of seafood provide the antioxidant vitamins C and E, selenium and zinc, which help to transport nutrients to the skin and maintain collagen and elastin levels. Zinc-rich foods, such as liver, pate and eggs, can improve conditions such as psoriasis and eczema.

Apples are rich in pectin, which helps to cleanse the liver, thus aiding detoxification of the skin.

Artichokes are good liver cleansers, too, along with asparagus and raw beetroot (beet). Fish, meat and eggs provide B vitamins, which promote a glowing complexion and combat dryness. Similar benefits are to be gained from eating oily fish such as mackerel, salmon, tuna, sardines and herrings. The fatty acids these fish contain (also found in nuts, seeds and vegetable oils) soften and hydrate the skin.

▼ A GLASS OF WATER WITH YOUR MEAL AIDS DIGESTION AND BENEFITS THE SKIN.

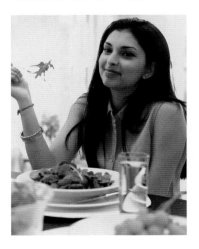

Cleansing avocados

These delicious fruits are renowned for their skin-kindly properties, mainly because of their high vitamin E content. Combined with parsley, asparagus and orange, this juice makes a great cleanser and skin tonic. As well as providing antioxidants, the presence of the citrus juices stops the avocado blend from discolouring, which means that it will keep in the refrigerator for a little while. If you find the blend becomes too thick for your taste, simply dilute with a small amount of mineral water.

▼ THIS CLEANSING AVOCADO BLEND IS LESS EXPENSIVE THAN MANY SKIN PRODUCTS. POUR OVER ICE CUBES TO SERVE, IF YOU LIKE.

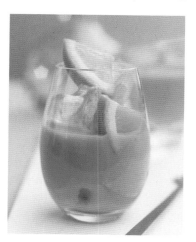

RECIPE SUGGESTION

Green devil

This blend makes two glasses, so you can save one for later.

Ingredients

1 small avocado

75g/3oz asparagus spears

small handful of parsley, tough stalks removed

2 large oranges

squeeze of lemon juice

orange wedges, to decorate

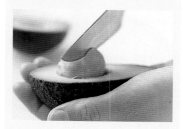

1 Halve the avocado and discard the stone (pit). Scoop the flesh into a blender or food processor. Roughly chop the asparagus and add to the avocado with the parsley. Blend thoroughly.

2 Juice the oranges and add to the mixture with the lemon juice. Blend again until smooth and even, then pour into a glass. Decorate with orange wedges.

Healthier nails

Our nails reveal quite a lot about our state of health. Ideally, they should be strong, well shaped and flexible. The nail bed should be pale pink, indicating that the blood is adequately oxygenated.

The best way to ensure nails are strong and healthy is to eat a balanced diet, with plenty of fresh fruit and vegetables.

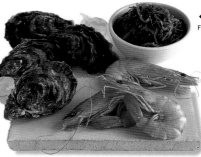

◀ SEAWEED AND SHELL-FISH CONTAIN ZINC.

so a meal of braised liver with onions and cherry tomatoes once a week may work wonders. Chickpeas and tofu are a good choice for vegetarians. It used to be thought that drinking milk – or eating cheese – was good for nails, because of the calcium these foods deliver, but this is inaccurate. Nails are made of a protein called keratin and contain little calcium.

Drink lots of water, and make sure that you get enough iron, which helps to prevent the nails from thinning. Foods that are good sources of iron include liver and other red meat, fish, poultry, green leafy vegetables, dried apricots, prunes and wholegrain cereals. To optimize iron absorption, eat suitable foods with ingredients that deliver vitamin C, such as tomatoes or potatoes, or drink orange juice with your meal. Avoid drinking tea, as the tannin impairs iron absorption.

If your nails are dry and brittle, you may not be getting enough zinc. Seafood (especially oysters), eggs and liver are good sources,

Wide ridges on the nails can indicate a deficiency of selenium, which is closely associated with the function of vitamin E in the body. Good sources are meat, especially liver, fish and shellfish, chicken and wholegrain cereals. Don't worry if you find little white spots on your nails – these are not sinister, and probably indicate minor damage, such as knocking against a table.

Seafood salvation

Shellfish work wonders for nails, thanks to the powerful combination of protein, zinc and vitamin E they provide. Mussels in particular are very easy to prepare – and the simplest cooking methods are often the best. Be sure to clean them thoroughly before simmering, by scrubbing the shells with plenty of cold water. Mussels should always be cooked with the shells closed, so give any obstinate ones a sharp tap. If they still refuse to close, simply discard them altogether. Finally, pull out and discard the fibrous 'beard' that sprouts between the two halves of the shell.

▾ Barnacles sometimes attach themselves to mussels; simply scrub the shells before cooking to remove.

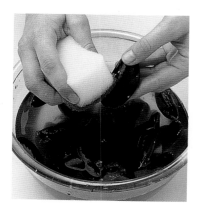

Anxiety and stress

It is almost impossible to avoid stress. A hectic workplace, unrealistic demands on our time, trying to juggle a job and care for a family, facing a life change such as retirement – all these elements make it increasingly difficult to cope.

If you are severely stressed, it is all too easy to bottle it up. Counselling can be beneficial or you may need medication. There are also some simple ways you can help yourself. A nutrient-rich diet combined with regular exercise and a healthy lifestyle can help to reduce anxiety levels. Your diet should include wholegrains, dairy products, liver, green vegetables, seafood, lean meat, nuts, seeds, yeast extract, pulses (legumes), eggs and fortified breakfast cereals. These are all good sources of B vitamins, which help the body cope with stressful situations, and correct poor sleep patterns. Vitamin C is depleted in times of stress, so eat citrus fruit, kiwi fruit, broccoli, potatoes and green leafy vegetables. Magnesium levels may be low, too: wholegrain cereals, nuts, pulses, sesame seeds, sea vegetables, dried figs and leafy green vegetables can help to restore the balance. Eating oily fish can also be beneficial, especially if you include the bones. This delivers a double benefit: omega-3 fatty acids and calcium for efficient functioning of the nerves.

Being stressed can affect health in many different ways. The most immediate, and obvious, is its effect on digestion. Taking time over meals, making sure you are relaxed when eating, eating a balanced diet with plenty of fresh fruit and vegetables, and drinking lots of water can only help.

▲ SARDINES ARE A HEALTHY OILY FISH.

RECIPE SUGGESTION

LENTIL AND TOMATO SOUP

This vegetable soup is one of the most comforting dishes of its kind. It is quick to make, as the lentils do not require any soaking beforehand. It works well as a nourishing lunch or end-of-day soother. Serves four.

INGREDIENTS

275g/10 oz/1¼ cups brown
*   lentils*
150ml/¼ pint/⅔ cup extra
*   virgin olive oil*
1 onion, thinly sliced
2 garlic cloves, sliced
1 carrot, sliced
400g/14oz can chopped
*   tomatoes*
15ml/1 tbsp tomato purée
*   (paste)*
2.5ml/½ tsp dried oregano
1 litre/1¾ pints/4 cups hot water
salt and ground black pepper
30ml/2 tbsp roughly chopped
*   fresh herbs to garnish*

1 Rinse and drain the lentils, put them in a large pan, and cover with cold water. Bring to the boil and boil for 3–4 minutes. Strain and set aside.

2 Sauté the sliced onion in the olive oil until translucent. Stir in the garlic and, as soon as it becomes aromatic, return the lentils to the pan. Add the carrot, tomatoes, tomato purée and oregano. Stir in the hot water and a little pepper.

3 Bring to the boil, then lower the heat, cover the pan and cook gently for 20–30 minutes.

4 Swirling the soup with a spoon should indicate whether it is ready to serve – the lentils should feel soft but should not have begun to disintegrate. Season and sprinkle with the chopped herbs before serving.

▼ THE SECRET OF A GOOD LENTIL SOUP IS TO ADD A GENEROUS MEASURE OF OLIVE OIL TO THE PAN BEFORE COOKING THE VEGETABLES IN STEP 2.

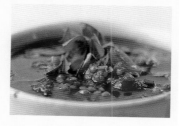

Minor depression

It is no coincidence that we crave sweet foods when we are feeling down. Studies show that sweet, carbohydrate foods, like biscuits, chocolate and cakes, help in the production of seratonin, a neurotransmitter that is said to lift the spirits.

Bingeing on sugary foods affects blood sugar levels, and a quick high will soon be followed by a deep low. The answer is to eat complex carbohydrates, like wholemeal (whole-wheat) bread, muffins or scones, cereal bars, brown rice or wholemeal pasta, which are broken down slowly in the body. They will give you a seratonin lift, but its effects will be even and last longer.

The amino acid tryptophan, which the body converts to seratonin, is found in lean meat, poultry, eggs, soya beans and some other pulses (legumes), dried dates, broccoli, low-fat dairy products, bananas and watercress, so next time you are feeling just a bit blue, chop up a banana with a couple of dried dates and eat it with a spoonful of low-fat yogurt. Sprinkle over a few Brazil nuts and you add selenium, a mood enhancer.

Not getting enough iron can lead to mild depression, so make sure you are getting enough of this valuable mineral, remembering that vitamin C is needed if the body is to absorb it properly.

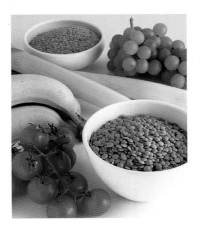

◀ FRUIT, PULSES (LEGUMES) AND VEGETABLES HELP TO KEEP BLOOD SUGAR LEVELS STABLE.

QUICK LIFT
Chillies stimulate the brain to release endorphins, which naturally boost the spirits. Ginger has a similar effect, so a meal of stir-fried chicken, liver or tofu with fresh root ginger and chillies is a savoury solution to feast upon if you are feeling down.

Broccoli and mushroom salad with tofu

This nutrient-packed salad is the ultimate remedy for a low mood. As well as boasting stimulating superfoods like broccoli, garlic and ginger, it also offers natural mood enhancers such as tofu, nuts and seeds. Serves four.

Ingredients

250g/9oz firm tofu, cubed
250g/9oz broccoli florets
15ml/1 tbsp olive oil
1 garlic clove, finely chopped
350g/12oz brown cap (cremini) mushrooms, sliced
4 spring onions (scallions), thinly sliced
75g/3oz/¾ cup pine nuts, toasted

For the marinade

1 garlic clove, crushed
2.5cm/1in piece fresh root ginger, finely grated
45ml/3 tbsp soy sauce
45ml/3 tbsp tamari soy sauce
45ml/3 tbsp dry sherry
1.5ml/¼ tsp cumin seeds, toasted and coarsely crushed
1.5ml/¼ tsp caster (superfine) sugar

1 Prepare the marinade by stirring all the ingredients together in a bowl. Add the tofu cubes and cook thoroughly, then leave to marinate for at least 1 hour. Steam the broccoli for about 4–5 minutes until tender, then drain.

2 Heat the oil and stir-fry the garlic over a low heat for 1 minute. Add the mushrooms and fry them over a high heat for 4–5 minutes until cooked. Add to the broccoli and season.

3 Toss the marinated tofu and any remaining marinade with the broccoli, mushrooms and spring onions. Sprinkle with the pine nuts and serve immediately.

▼ THE QUANTITY OF ALCOHOL USED IN THE MARINADE IS FAIRLY SMALL, BUT YOU CAN OMIT IT ALTOGETHER IF YOU PREFER.

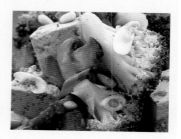

Healthy comfort foods

There is little doubt about the comforts of eating good food, but eating the wrong kind in a moment of need can only add to the burden of bad feeling. Choose light, nourishing snacks to enhance well-being and rekindle positive thoughts.

The healthiest comfort foods are often small, simple and familiar. Childhood treats such as boiled eggs with toasted bread soldiers or warming, satisfying soups inspire feelings of security at times of emotional upheaval, and ward off the temptation to seek out a quick sugar fix. Not that sweeter-tasting snacks are altogether bad: proper custard made with eggs is really quite nutritious, and baked egg custards are wonderful served with fruit for an added boost of Vitamin C. You can also try chunky sandwiches filled with fruity jam or mashed bananas with a sprinkling of cinnamon. Both of these will help energy levels to rise and ward off inertia or low spirits.

Some foods just make you feel wide awake and full of energy. Fresh flavours, zesty seasonings and a bit of colour work wonders. Opt for uplifting drinks to go with simple snacks or a bowl of breakfast cereal – try fresh fruit and vegetable juices, smoothies that are packed full of nutrients, and fresh fruit shakes. Use herbs and spices that are enlivening – sunny basil and head-clearing mint are good with savoury snacks.

When the body needs energy, go for fruit, pulses (legumes), wholemeal (whole-wheat) bread and pasta, all of which will slowly release energy into the bloodstream, ensuring long-term recovery. This is particularly important after any form of exercise that leaves the muscles depleted of energy.

▼ PORRIDGE AND STEWED FRUITS HELP TO SUSTAIN ENERGY LEVELS THROUGH THE DAY.

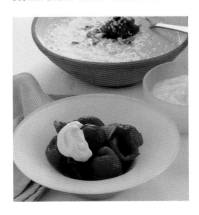

REAL CUSTARD

Although readily available in instant form, there is just no denying the joy of real custard. This classic version is enriched with egg and needs relatively little sugar to sweeten it, thanks to the addition of vanilla extract. Enjoy it with all kinds of heart-warming puddings!

INGREDIENTS

450ml/¾ pint/scant 2 cups milk

few drops of vanilla extract

2 eggs plus 1 egg yolk

15–30ml/1–2 tbsp caster (superfine) sugar

15ml/1 tbsp cornflour (cornstarch)

30ml/2 tbsp water

1 Heat the milk in a pan with the vanilla extract and remove from the heat just as the milk comes to the boil.

2 Whisk the eggs and yolk in a bowl with the caster sugar until well combined but not frothy. In a separate bowl, blend together the cornflour with the water and mix into the eggs. Whisk in a little of the hot milk, then mix in all the remaining milk.

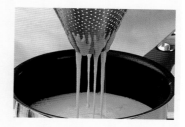

3 Strain the egg and milk mixture back into the pan and heat gently, stirring frequently. Take care not to overheat the mixture or it will curdle.

4 Continue stirring until the custard is thick enough to coat the back of a wooden spoon. Do not boil. Serve immediately.

▼ IT'S WELL WORTH TAKING THE TIME TO PREPARE REAL CUSTARD.

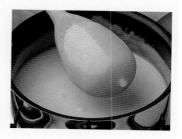

Diabetes

The incidence of diabetes in the Western world is increasing. Many cases of the milder form of this disease are not diagnosed, or are diagnosed too late to prevent some lasting damage, so it is important to be aware of the symptoms.

Diabetes is the result of the body's inability to control the amount of glucose in the blood. An essential form of energy, glucose is produced when we digest starchy and sugary foods. Blood glucose levels rise until a certain level is reached, whereupon the pancreas releases insulin to bring the levels back to normal. If the pancreas fails to produce insulin, Type 1 – insulin-dependent diabetes – is the result. If the body fails to utilize insulin correctly, or the pancreas becomes inefficient, Type 2 – sometimes referred to as adult-onset diabetes – occurs. Symptoms of untreated diabetes include thirst, frequent urination, headaches, blurred vision, weight-loss or nausea.

All diabetics need to control their diet with professional help. To keep blood sugar levels under control, it is vital to eat a balanced, healthy diet, and to lose any excess weight under medical supervision. The diet should be high in high-fibre, starchy carbohydrates, which raise blood glucose levels gradually and maintain them for longer. Wholemeal (whole-wheat) bread, potatoes, rice and pasta are recommended. It is important to eat five portions of vegetables and fruit daily, but very sweet fruit should only be eaten occasionally, because of the fructose they contain. Diabetics who are not overweight may be able to eat very small amounts of sugar in food, but

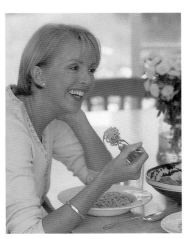

◀ EATING SMALL REGULAR MEALS WILL HELP KEEP YOUR BLOOD SUGAR LEVELS STEADY.

should avoid sweets and sweetened drinks. A low-fat diet is essential, as diabetics have an increased risk of coronary heart disease. Salt should be limited.

It is important to eat regular meals. Grazing – eating little and often – may be a good approach for Type 2 diabetics, helping to keep blood sugar levels steady.

QUICK BEAN FEAST RECIPE SUGGESTIONS

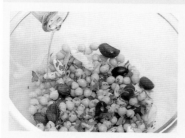

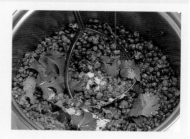

• Mix cooked chickpeas with spring onions (scallions), olives and chopped parsley, then drizzle over a little olive oil and some lemon juice.

• Mash cooked beans with olive oil, garlic and coriander (cilantro) and pile on to toasted wholemeal (whole-wheat) bread. Top with a poached egg.

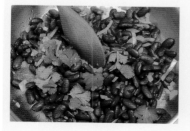

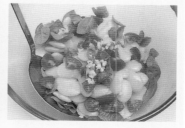

• Heat a little olive oil and stir-fry cooked red kidney beans with chopped onion, chilli, garlic and fresh coriander leaves.

• Dress cooked beans with extra virgin olive oil, lemon juice, crushed garlic, diced tomato and fresh basil.

Restless legs

This may sound like a puppet's problem. The syndrome usually occurs when you sit or lie down. The legs jerk involuntarily and there may be discomfort, "pins and needles" or a burning pain.

The problem is often at its worst at night, making it difficult for sufferers to get to sleep. The cause is unknown, but there is some evidence that RLS (restless leg syndrome) can be inherited. It can also begin at any age. Women who suffer from it may find their symptoms worsen when they are pregnant or in later years during the menopause.

It may help to choose a diet that is rich in iron. Liver, dried apricots, prunes and wholegrain cereals are good sources (avoid liver if you are pregnant). Folate, which is essential for building new body cells, can also ease the symptoms, so eat liver, pulses (legumes), green vegetables and wholegrain cereals. It is also worth increasing your intake of vitamin B12 by eating lean meat and dairy produce.

RLS may worsen as you age. It can be linked to circulatory problems, so the diet should include foods that are rich in vitamin E, such as avocados and beansprouts.

RECIPE SUGGESTION

SPICED APRICOT PURÉE
Try this with natural yogurt.

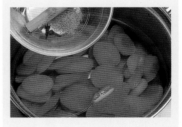

1 Place 350g/12oz/1½ cups dried apricots in a pan with water to cover. Add 1 cinnamon stick, 2 cloves and 2.5ml/½ tsp freshly grated nutmeg. Simmer until soft.

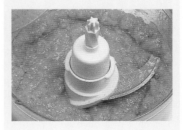

2 Remove the cinnamon stick and cloves. Leave to cool, then purée until smooth.

Fatigue

Are you often exhausted, too weary even to contemplate getting undressed for bed? Do you fall asleep at your desk after lunch? Have you been known to wake up feeling weary or as if you need a good night's sleep?

All the above are typical of chronic fatigue, which can be linked to a medical condition such as diabetes, and must be investigated by a doctor. General tiredness, however, is something all of us suffer from time to time. It may be unavoidable, the result of sleepless nights getting up to a small baby, or studying hard for an exam, or it may be linked to depression or a similar emotional state.

There may be a physical explanation, such as iron deficiency.

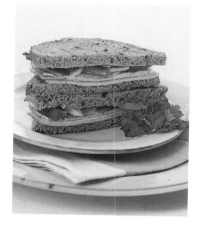

▲ COMPLEX CARBOHYDRATES PROVIDE AND SUSTAIN CONSTANT ENERGY LEVELS. CHOOSE BREADS CONTAINING WHOLEGRAINS.

ENERGIZE

If your energy levels have taken a dive because your blood sugar is low, don't reach for a bar of chocolate or a rich biscuit. The quick energy boost these give will be followed by a slump, and you may end up far more tired than you were at the start. Eat a wholemeal (whole-wheat) salad sandwich instead; the carbohydrate in the bread will give you a more efficient energy fix that will be more prolonged and even.

This can happen when a woman has particularly heavy periods. To redress the balance, eat iron-rich foods such as dried apricots, liver, red meat, pulses (legumes), eggs, green leafy vegetables, fortified breakfast cereals, seeds and wholegrains. At the same time, eat citrus fruit, kiwi fruit or blackcurrants. These are good sources of vitamin C, which is necessary for the uptake of iron into the bloodstream.

The morning after

A few drinks in the company of friends provide a welcome tonic to the stresses of life, but if enjoyed to excess you may feel pretty rotten the next day. Food is a great healer, however, and the right kind will soon get you back on track.

Having a hangover is the classic comfort-food zone. For the worst cases, plain toast, porridge and cereals with milk are a good choice. Breakfast cereals that are fortified with B-group vitamins are good for replenishing supplies when absorption has been inhibited by alcohol. Fruit in yogurt is refreshing and nutritious – bananas are easy to digest, and low-fat yogurt with honey works wonders. Pears are light in flavour, easy to digest and not too disruptive. Papaya, mango, kiwi and orange all provide useful antioxidant vitamins.

Intense hunger often accompanies a modest hangover. A hearty cooked brunch works wonders, if eaten a few hours after waking up. Grilled tomatoes and bacon, poached or scrambled eggs, mushrooms and plenty of warm crusty bread might all appeal. If cooking is too much trouble, cooked ham or finely sliced cheese served in wholemeal rolls is plain, comforting and instantly satisfying fare.

Semi-sweet breads, such as currant buns or brioche, or American muffins with fresh and dried fruit and bran are a perfect choice. Blueberry muffins are refreshing, and they go well with bananas in yogurt.

The following page features two brilliantly simple but extremely effective hangover cures.

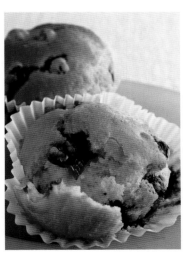

◀ HOME-BAKED MUFFINS ARE A DELICIOUS START TO A HANGOVER DAY. IF YOU CANNOT FACE COOKING, BUY THEM FRESH.

Bacon sandwich

These snacks provide vitamins, minerals and oodles of soothing familiarity – use either chunky back bacon or thin crispy rashers (slices). This will make two cut sandwiches or rolls.

Ingredients

8 bacon rashers

2 crisp fresh rolls or 4 thick
   slices of toast, buttered

Small bunch of spring onions
   (scallions)

a little ketchup or brown sauce

Grill (broil) or fry the bacon to taste. Spread a little sauce on the buttered toast or roll halves, place the cooked bacon between them and serve at once. Add sliced avocado or grilled red (bell) pepper slices for antioxidant vitamins to counteract the effects of the alcohol.

Prairie oyster

This is an alcohol-free version of a classic 'hair of the dog' drink usually served with a large measure of spirits.

Ingredients

25ml/1½ tbsp cider vinegar

25ml/1½ tbsp Worcestershire
   sauce

5ml/1 tsp tomato ketchup

5ml/1 tsp Angostura bitters

dash of tabasco

1 raw egg yolk

1 Mix all the ingredients except the egg yolk in a glass, then slide in the egg yolk, taking care not to break it. Do not stir. Down the mixture in one gulp.

▼ Raw egg provides a useful shot of protein. Use an organic, free-range egg to minimize health risks.

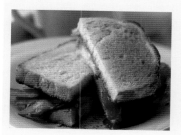

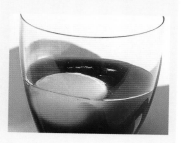

Joint problems

Aching joints are a common problem, especially as we get older. The condition may be related to a recognized medical condition, such as rheumatoid arthritis or osteoarthritis, but may simply be down to general wear and tear.

Whatever the cause, aching joints are no fun. Simply straightening up or getting in and out of a car can be very uncomfortable. There is a lot of discussion as to whether diet has any role to play in the prevention or treatment of either condition, but several recent studies suggest that antioxidants and oily fish may help.

▼ DOING TOO MUCH GARDENING, OR TAKING UNACCUSTOMED EXERCISE CAN MAKE YOUR JOINTS STIFF AND UNCOMFORTABLE.

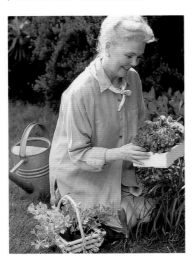

ARTHRITIS

The most common forms of this condition are rheumatoid arthritis and osteoarthritis. The former is a complex condition whose cause is largely unknown. It is an inflammatory condition affecting the joints and is thought to be related to a malfunctioning immune system. It can strike at any age. Osteoarthritis is a degenerative condition of the joints, which most commonly occurs with age, and tends to affect those who are overweight. Certain foods may bring relief to arthritis sufferers, but others can make the symptoms worse. If this happens, an allergy may be implicated. Consult an expert, who may recommend you try an exclusion diet, followed by a tailor-made diet plan.

You can boost your antioxidant intake by eating plenty of green leafy vegetables, also carrots, broccoli, sweet potatoes and avocados, which contain appreciable amounts of vitamins C and E, betacarotene and selenium. Apricots, apples,

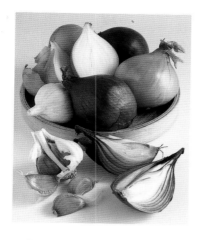

▲ ONIONS ARE ONE OF THE OLDEST NATURAL CURES. THEY STIMULATE THE BODY'S ANTIOXIDANT MECHANISMS AND HELP ARTHRITIS, RHEUMATISM AND GOUT.

sufferers and may help those with osteoarthritis. It is certainly worth eating oily fish more often (about three times a week is recommended) as there are other health benefits too. The vitamin B12 in oily fish is important for a healthy nervous system, and the iodine promotes healthy thyroid function. Fish oils are rich in omega-3 fatty acids, which can help to reduce inflammation. Vegetarians should eat soya beans, tofu, linseeds, wheatgerm, walnuts and rapeseed oil: all good alternative sources of omega-3 fatty acids.

bananas and mangoes are the best fruits to eat. Try eating asparagus and celery, both of which have anti-inflammatory properties, and may help to reduce swelling and ease painful joints. Another anti-inflammatory agent is quercetin, which is found in kelp, onions and apples. Spices that have anti-inflammatory qualities include turmeric and fresh root ginger.

EAT MORE OILY FISH

Salmon, tuna, mackerel, sardines and herrings have been shown to offer relief to rheumatoid arthritis

ASPARAGUS HEALER

Try a simple egg-lemon sauce with boiled asparagus. Boil a small bundle (tough ends removed) in salted water for 7–10 minutes. Reserve the cooking juices and blend with about 15ml/1tbsp cornflour (cornstarch) until the sauce thickens. Remove from the heat and stir in about 10ml/2tsp sugar. Cool. Beat two egg yolks with the juice of 1½ lemons and gradually stir into the cooled sauce. Drizzle a little sauce over the cooked asparagus and chill the dish, and remaining sauce, for at least two hours before serving.

Women's health

Fluctuating hormone levels have a marked effect on women's well-being. Balance can be easier to achieve if you adopt a healthy lifestyle, enjoy plenty of regular exercise and watch what you eat.

PRE-MENSTRUAL SYNDROME (PMS)

Any woman who regularly experiences pre-menstrual syndrome (PMS) will need no explanation of the symptoms. Mood swings, irritability, food cravings, bloating, constipation and diarrhoea can all occur, and when these symptoms are every month, 2–14 days before a period starts, life can be difficult.

Certain foods may offer some benefits. Wheatgerm, wholegrains, bananas, oily fish and poultry are

▼ TAKING PLENTY OF EXERCISE AND EATING A BALANCED DIET WILL HELP RELIEVE PMS.

good sources of vitamin B6, which is especially helpful in combating water retention and breast tenderness. Vitamin B6 can aid the absorption of magnesium, a lack of which causes mood swings and cravings. Magnesium is found in fruits and vegetables. Jacket potatoes (with the skin) are an excellent source, as are avocados and Chinese leaves (Chinese cabbage). Dried apricots, liver, red meat, eggs, green leafy vegetables, seeds and wholegrains are rich in iron, a lack of which can lead to anaemia and

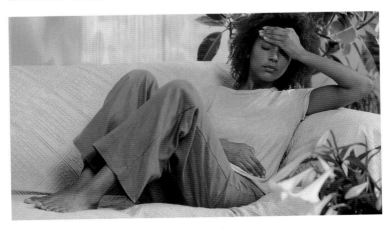

fatigue. To help the body absorb iron, take in plenty of vitamin C, such as kiwi fruit and blackcurrants.

Breast pain can cause discomfort. It may be eased by eating foods rich in essential fatty acids such as oily fish, sunflower oil, rapeseed oil, nuts and seeds, or by eating foods rich in vitamin E such as vegetable oils, nuts, avocados, eggs and wheatgerm.

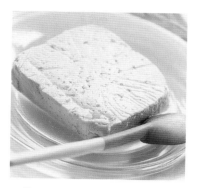

▲ TOFU IS AVAILABLE IN DIFFERENT FORMS, AND CAN BE USED IN SOUPS, SALADS AND STIR-FRIES.

MENOPAUSE

Some women sail through the menopause, but others experience side effects, such as depression, insomnia and anxiety, hot flushes, vaginal dryness and night sweats. These symptoms can be eased by HRT (hormone replacement therapy), but a healthy diet may help.

There is current interest in the role of phytoestrogens – chemicals in plants that act in a similar way to the female hormone, oestrogen. Japanese women, whose diets are high in phytoestrogens, have few menopausal problems and a lower risk of breast cancer. It is hoped that trials will confirm whether eating more phytoestrogen-rich food – soya beans, tofu, soy milk and linseeds – can help Western women.

It is believed that soya products may help to maintain bone density and also reduce the risk of breast cancer. Sweet potatoes contain natural progesterone, and may help to correct hormone imbalance and ease menopausal symptoms. To slow down bone density loss during menopause, eat calcium-rich foods like low-fat dairy products, nuts, seeds, green leafy vegetables, canned fish, pulses, seaweed and bread. Foods rich in vitamin D, zinc and magnesium are also valuable.

Treat yourself to an avocado now and then. This vegetable is rich in potassium, which helps to prevent fluid retention, and is high in vitamin E, which may help to alleviate hot flushes.

The following recipes are perfect antidotes to time-of-the-month blues or the symptoms that often signal hormonal change. They are easy to prepare, have the right combination of B-vitamins and restorative minerals, and that comfort factor too! Serve them as snacks, lunches or as side-dishes to a main meal.

Potatoes, like certain other fruits, root vegetables and seeds, are an important source of estrogen, which can help during the menopause. Other vegetables will actually inhibit estrogen, however, and this can be of interest to those suffering symptoms connected with PMS. Consult a nutritional expert to learn more about the foods that perform these functions.

▼ POTATOES ARE HEALTHIEST COOKED IN THEIR SKINS. TRY THEM DEEP-FRIED, SERVED WITH SPICY YOGURT DIP.

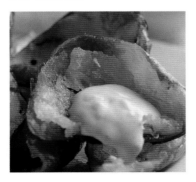

BAKED POTATO BLISS
For super-fast potatoes cooked in their skins, microwave on a high setting for 10–15 minutes.

DEEP-FRIED JACKETS WITH SPICY YOGURT DIP
First, prepare the dip. Blend 120ml/4fl oz/½ cup natural (plain) yogurt with a crushed garlic clove, 5ml/1 tsp tomato purée (paste), half a chopped green chilli and a sprinkling of salt. Chill while the potatoes are baking. When the baked potatoes are sufficiently cool, slice in half and scoop out the middle. Deep-fry the potato halves on both sides until golden-brown and serve with the dip.

BAKED POTATO SALAD
Remove the skins from the baked potatoes and cut into chunks, then toss with 50ml/2 fl oz/¼ cup white wine vinegar, 75ml/5 tbsp olive oil and 30ml/ 2 tbsp chopped flat leaf parsley. Add a handful each of capers and olives, and top with marinated anchovies.

Smoked salmon pancakes with pine nuts

An excellent way to dose up on important fatty acids, these sumptuous little pancakes take just minutes to make. Alternatively, if you suffer from bloating around the time of your period, or if you have a gluten intolerance, prepare a simple, healthy snack of wheat-free oat cakes topped with the smoked salmon and crème fraiche or sour cream.

INGREDIENTS

120ml/4fl oz/½ cup milk
115g/4oz/1 cup self-raising (self-rising) flour
1 egg
30ml/2 tbsp pesto
vegetable oil, for frying
200ml/7fl oz/scant 1 cup crème fraîche or sour cream
75g/3oz smoked salmon
15ml/1 tbsp pine nuts, toasted
salt and ground black pepper
fresh basil, to garnish

1 Pour half the milk into a mixing bowl. Beat in the flour, egg and pesto and mix thoroughly to make a smooth batter.

2 Add the remainder of the milk and mix until evenly blended.

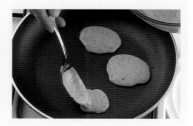

3 Heat the vegetable oil and spoon the batter into small heaps. Allow about 30 seconds for the pancakes to cook, then turn and cook briefly on the other side.

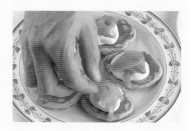

4 Arrange the pancakes on a serving plate and top each one with a spoonful of crème fraîche or sour cream. Cut the salmon into pieces to fit the top of the pancakes and lightly place them on top of the cream. Top with pine nuts and fresh basil.

A healthy heart

What you eat has a direct bearing on the health and efficiency of your heart and circulation. You may not be able to do anything about hereditary heart disease or stroke, but you can eat sensibly, take exercise and avoid obesity.

Reducing the amount of saturated fat you consume is a vital first step. Limit dairy products, fatty meat and hydrogenated or trans fats found in margarine and processed foods. Foods high in saturated fats are chocolates, cakes, sauces, biscuits (cookies) and puddings. Saturated fat may be listed as hydrogenated vegetable fat or oil.

Eat plenty of fresh fruit and vegetables. The fibre, phytochemicals, antioxidants and vitamins they

▼ EATING FOODS HIGH IN VITAMIN E CAN HELP TO IMPROVE THE CIRCULATORY SYSTEM.

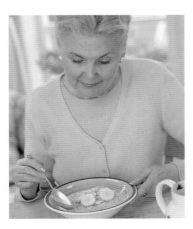

contribute help to prevent the blocking of the arteries. Green, leafy vegetables and pulses (legumes) are high in folate, which reduces levels of homocysteine. This amino acid has been linked to increased risk of coronary heart disease and strokes. Eat one or two garlic cloves a day. Garlic has been found to lower blood cholesterol levels, reduce blood pressure and help to prevent blood clots forming.

Omega-3 oils have the same effect. You'll find these in oily fish, walnuts, wheatgerm and soya beans. Just one serving of oily fish a week is believed to cut the risk of heart attack by half.

Eat oats, lentils, nuts and pulses. The insoluble fibre they contain can reduce blood cholesterol levels when eaten as part of a low-fat diet.

Red wine, tea and onions all contain the flavonoid quercetin, which may reduce the risk of heart disease and strokes. Drink wine in moderation only.

THERAPEUTIC GARLIC

Garlic has always been regarded as a useful aid to the body's ability to fight infection, but medical research has also proved that it can help to lower blood pressure and reduce cholesterol, making it a particularly useful dietary tool against heart disease. It's so easy to incorporate garlic into a healthy, balanced diet. Add chopped garlic to sauces, soups and pâtés, or blend it with butter or oil to drizzle over breads and baked vegetables.

GREAT GARLIC RECIPE SUGGESTIONS

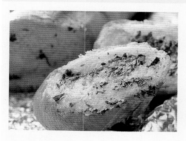

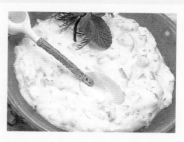

• Roast two or three garlic cloves, remove the skins when cool and crush with softened butter and a pinch of herbs. Spread between a split loaf and bake in foil.

• Soak a couple of white bread slices in milk, then process to a coarse paste with a few garlic cloves, peeled and chopped, a handful of shelled walnuts and a drizzle each of olive and walnut oils. Add a squeeze of lemon juice to taste, dust with paprika and serve as a nutty-textured sauce.

• Crush and blend a couple of garlic cloves with thick natural (plain) yogurt, diced cucumber and chopped fresh dill and mint for a cooling dip for a spicy dish.

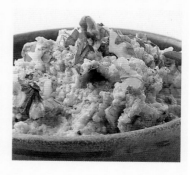

Boosting the immune system

A healthy immune system is the key to maintaining general good health and keeping infections at bay. Poor diet and stress have a negative effect on the immune system, leaving the body vulnerable to colds, flu and disease.

A diet based on unprocessed foods, along with a healthy lifestyle, is essential for maintaining the immune system. Raw fruits and vegetables, especially sprouting seeds, are particularly helpful.

Key protective foods include good sources of the antioxidant vitamins C and E, and betacarotene, which help to boost the immune system. Sweet potatoes and avocados are ideal, as are berry fruit (especially blackcurrants) and citrus fruit. Limes and lemons are also good for colds, coughs and sore throats, and have potent antiseptic properties.

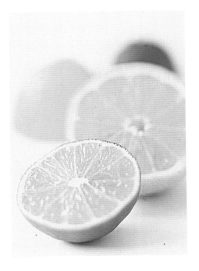

▲ Citrus fruits are a rich source of vitamin C.

Pumpkin seeds

Boost your zinc intake with pumpkin seeds by
• Sprinkling them over baked goods before cooking.
• Adding them to flapjacks.
• Tossing them into a stir-fry.
• Adding them to a sweet crumble topping.
• Using them to make pesto.
• Scattering them over a salad.

Also good are wholegrains, meat, tuna, salmon, nuts, dried fruits, seeds and bananas, which provide vitamin B. This supports the body's production of antibodies. Zinc is an essential mineral to boost and support a healthy immune system. It can be found in shellfish such as oysters and crab, eggs, beef, turkey, pumpkin seeds, peanuts, cheese and yogurt.

FRUIT AND NUT FLAPJACKS
This chewy combination of nuts, seeds and dried fruit makes a sweet but nutritious treat.

INGREDIENTS
150g/5oz/⅔ cup unsalted (sweet) butter, diced
150g/5oz/⅔ cup light muscovado (brown) sugar
30ml/2 tbsp maple syrup
200g/7oz/2 cups rolled oats
50g/2oz/½ cup pecan nuts, chopped
50g/2oz/¼ cup ready-to-eat dried apricots, chopped

1 Preheat the oven to 160°C/ 325°F/Gas 3. Lightly grease an 18cm/7in square shallow baking tin (pan). Put the butter, sugar and maple syrup in a large heavy pan and heat gently until the butter has melted. Remove from the heat and stir in the oats, nuts and apricots until these have been well combined.

2 Spread evenly in the prepared tin and, using a knife, score the mixture into ten bars. Bake for 25–30 minutes until golden.

PESTO WITH PUMPKIN SEEDS
Substituting the traditional pine nuts with toasted pumpkin seeds offers a welcome twist on the classic pesto recipe.

INGREDIENTS
50g/2oz fresh basil leaves
25g/1oz/¼ cup pumpkin seeds, toasted
2 garlic cloves, peeled
120ml/4 fl oz/½ cup olive oil
25g/1oz/⅓ cup fresh Parmesan cheese, grated

Process the basil leaves to a paste with the toasted seeds and garlic cloves. With the motor still running, drizzle in the olive oil until the mixture forms a paste. Spoon into a bowl, stir in the Parmesan, and season to taste with a sprinkling of freshly ground black pepper.

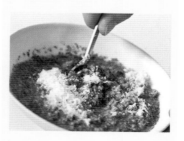

Food allergy and intolerance

Food does not always heal. Food sensitivities – allergies and intolerances – seem to be on the increase, and can cause anything from minor discomfort to more serious risk in susceptible individuals.

An allergic reaction is not the same as a food intolerance. The former occurs when the body reacts to an essentially harmless substance as though it were an invading organism like a bacterium. An immune response is triggered and antibodies are activated to deal with the threat. What happens next depends on the individual, the site of the problem and the allergen itself.

Sneezing and watering eyes are common, as are hives, asthma and eczema. Sometimes the reaction is violent, and can be life threatening, as is the case with peanut allergy.

Food intolerance is more subtle, occurring when the body finds a substance difficult to cope with. Why this should happen is not always clear, but when the offending food is located and omitted

▼ TRY TO ELIMINATE ONE FOOD AT A TIME FROM YOUR DIET AND NOTE ANY CHANGES.

▼ AN ORANGE JUICE ALLERGY DOESN'T MEAN YOU CAN'T EAT OTHER CITRUS FRUITS.

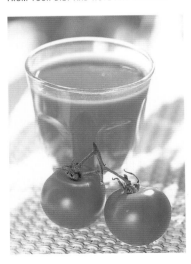

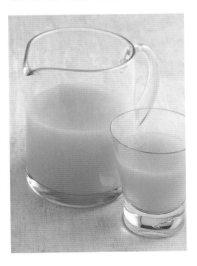

from the diet, the results can be quite dramatic.

There are many different types of food intolerance. Among the common culprits are soya products, caffeine, chocolate, orange juice, tomatoes and food additives. The lactose in cow's milk and the gluten in wheat, rye and barley are often implicated. The symptoms are wide ranging, but can include anxiety, depression, fatigue, headaches, skin disorders, asthma, joint or muscle pain, rheumatoid arthritis and mouth or stomach ulcers. Irritable bowel syndrome can be linked to a food intolerance.

It is one thing to suspect a food allergy or intolerance; quite another to track it down. Seek advice from a doctor, dietician or naturopath.

ALTERNATIVES

If you are lactose intolerant, try switching to soya milk, but make sure you get sufficient calcium from other sources. Live yogurt can often be tolerated, as the bacteria in the yogurt helps to break down the lactose.

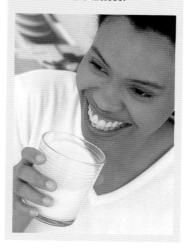

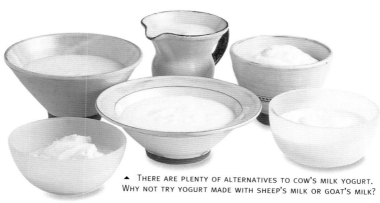

▲ THERE ARE PLENTY OF ALTERNATIVES TO COW'S MILK YOGURT. WHY NOT TRY YOGURT MADE WITH SHEEP'S MILK OR GOAT'S MILK?

Glossary

Amino acids These are the basic components of proteins. There are 20 in all, 12 of which can be synthesized by the body and eight which must come from our food.

▲ OYSTERS

Quinoa, pronounced "keen-wa", is the only known complete food, in that it contains all eight of the essential amino acids that the body cannot make. Usually our bodies obtain them from a variety of foods.

Antioxidants Found in vitamins A, C and E, in co-enzyme Q10 and betacarotene, as well as in minerals like selenium and zinc, these help to mop up free radicals in the body, thus limiting tissue damage.

Betacarotene is what gives fruit and vegetables such as mangoes, apricots, carrots, (bell) peppers and sweet potatoes their bright orange colour. An important antioxidant, betacarotene can be converted into vitamin A by the body.

Carcinogens are cancer-causing substances.

Complex carbohydrates These are contained in fresh fruit, wholemeal (whole-wheat) bread, fruit bread, wholemeal muffins or scones, wholegrain cereal, brown rice and wholemeal or buckwheat pasta. The body breaks complex carbohydrates down slowly, providing sustained energy over a long period of time. Complex carbohydrates can also promote sleep if they are eaten towards the end of the day.

Enzymes These are protein molecules that act as catalysts in the body, making it possible for biological processes to take place. Metabolic enzymes are implicated in the building of healthy bones, tissues and muscle. Digestive enzymes, most of which come from the food we eat, ensure that food is digested and made available to the body, or eliminated. Enzymes are

▼ WALNUTS

vital for every biological function and poor enzyme activity can seriously damage our health.

Essential fatty acids Fatty acids are responsible for several bodily processes, including the maintenance of cell walls. The body can manufacture most fatty acids, but two main types – essential fatty acids – must come from food. These are omega-3, found in oily fish, walnuts and rapeseed oil; and omega-6, from corn oil and sunflower oil. These fats are "good" fats, and should be eaten regularly. In effect they help the body to process damaging fats.

Free radicals These are damaging molecules produced by the body as part of a natural process. The chemical structure of a free radical differs from a healthy molecule in that it has an unpaired electron. The electron roams the body searching for a healthy electron to pair up with. This process damages

▼ SWEET POTATOES

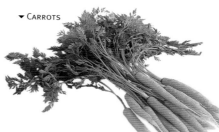
▼ CARROTS

the host molecule, changing its DNA irreversibly. Free radicals only survive for a short time, but if they exist in large numbers they can cause extensive cell damage resulting in heart disease, cataracts and cancer. Eating foods rich in antioxidants eliminates free radicals from the body.

Goitre is a painful swelling of the thyroid gland.

Phytochemicals are plant compounds, widely found in fruit and vegetables, which appear to offer protection against diseases like cancer, arthritis, heart disease and hypertension, and may slow down the ageing process. Phytochemicals also have antioxidant properties.

Phytoestrogens These are chemicals found in plants. They mimic the action of the female sex hormone, oestrogen, and can be helpful in reducing menopausal symptoms. Soya beans are a good source.

glossary **253**

Essential vitamins and minerals

VITAMIN	BEST SOURCES	ROLE IN HEALTH
A (retinol in animal foods, beta-carotene in plant foods)	Milk, butter, cheese, egg yolks and margarine, carrots, apricots, squash, red (bell) peppers, broccoli, green leafy vegetables, mango and sweet potatoes.	Essential for vision, bone growth and skin and tissue repair. Beta-carotene acts as an antioxidant and protects the immune system.
B1 (thiamin)	Wholegrain cereals, brewer's yeast, potatoes, nuts, pulses (legumes) and milk.	Essential for energy production, the nervous system, muscles and heart. Promotes growth and boosts mental ability.
B2 (riboflavin)	Cheese, eggs, milk, yogurt, fortified breakfast cereals, yeast extract, almonds and pumpkin seeds.	Essential for energy production and for the functioning of vitamin B6 and niacin as well as tissue repair.
Niacin (part of B complex)	Pulses, potatoes, fortified breakfast cereals, wheatgerm, peanuts, milk, cheese, eggs, peas, mushrooms, green leafy vegetables, figs and prunes.	Essential for healthy digestive system, skin and circulation. It is also needed for the release of energy.
B6 (piridoxine)	Eggs, wholemeal (whole-wheat) bread, breakfast cereals, nuts, bananas and cruciferous vegetables, such as broccoli and cabbage.	Essential for assimilating protein and fat, to make red blood cells, and a healthy immune system.
B12 (cyanocobalamin)	Milk, eggs, fortified breakfast cereals, cheese and yeast extract.	Essential for formation of red blood cells, maintaining a healthy nervous system and increasing energy levels.
Folate (folic acid)	Green leafy vegetables, fortified breakfast cereals, bread, nuts, pulses, bananas and yeast extract.	Essential for cell division. Extra is needed pre-conception and during pregnancy to protect foetus against neural tube defects.
C (ascorbic acid)	Citrus fruits, melons, strawberries, tomatoes, broccoli, potatoes, peppers and green vegetables.	Essential for the absorption of iron, healthy skin, teeth and bones. An antioxidant that strengthens bones.
D (calciferol)	Sunlight, margarine, vegetable oils, eggs, cereals and butter.	Essential for bone and teeth formation, helps the body to absorb calcium and phosphorus.
E (tocopherol)	Seeds, nuts, vegetable oils, eggs, wholemeal bread, green leafy vegetables, oats and cereals.	Essential for healthy skin, circulation and maintaining cells – an antioxidant.

MINERAL	BEST SOURCES	ROLE IN HEALTH
Calcium	Milk, cheese, yogurt, green leafy vegetables, sesame seeds, broccoli, dried figs, pulses, almonds, spinach and watercress.	Essential for building and maintaining bones and teeth, muscle function and the nervous system.
Iron	Egg yolks, fortified breakfast cereals, green leafy vegetables, dried apricots, prunes, pulses, wholegrains and tofu.	Essential for healthy blood and muscles.
Zinc	Peanuts, wholegrains sunflower and pumpkin seeds, pulses, milk, hard cheese and yogurt.	Essential for a healthy immune system, tissue formation, normal growth and wound healing and reproduction.
Sodium	Most salt we eat comes from processed foods such as crisps, cheese and canned foods. It is also found naturally in most foods.	Essential for nerve and muscle function and the regulation of body fluid.
Potassium	Bananas, milk, pulses, nuts, seeds, wholegrains, potatoes, fruits and vegetables.	Essential for water balance, normal blood pressure and nerve transmission.
Magnesium	Nuts, seeds, wholegrains, pulses, tofu, dried figs and apricots and vegetables.	Essential for healthy muscles, bones and teeth, normal growth and nerves.
Phosphorous	Milk, cheese, yogurt, eggs, nuts, seeds, pulses and wholegrains.	Essential for healthy bones and teeth, energy production and the assimilation of nutrients.
Selenium	Avocados, lentils, milk, cheese, butter, brazil nuts and seaweed.	Essential for protecting against free radical damage and may protect against cancer.
Iodine	Seaweed and iodized salt.	Aids the production of hormones released by the thyroid gland.
Chloride	Table salt and foods that contain salt.	Regulates and maintains the balance of fluids in the body.
Manganese	Nuts, wholegrains, pulses, tofu and tea.	Essential component of various enzymes that are involved in energy production.

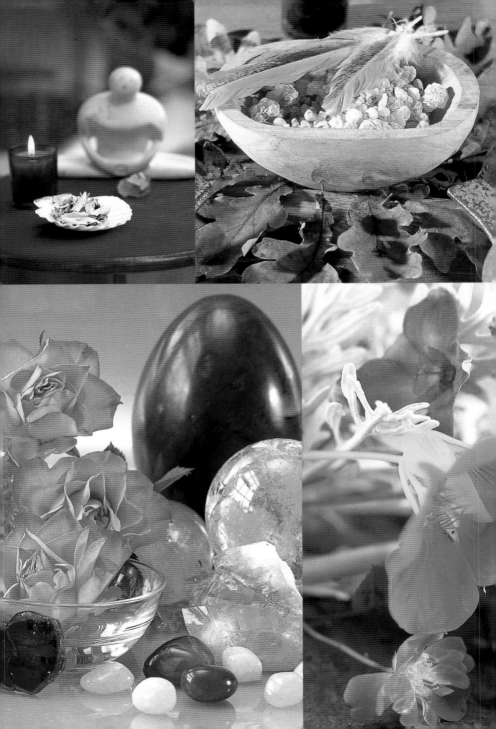

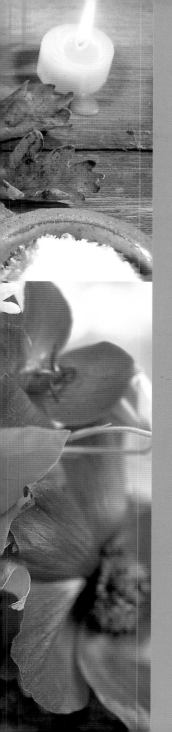

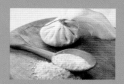

HEALING WITH
AYURVEDA

According to legend, the 52 great Rishis (seers) of ancient India discovered the Veda, or knowledge of how the universe works, in their meditations. These secrets were then organized into a system known as Ayurveda, which means "science of life".

Increasingly popular as a holistic system of healthcare in the West, Ayurveda gives clear instructions on how we can achieve physical and spiritual well-being. Through an understanding of our constitutional type, or dosha, it shows how we can prevent and treat disease by paying attention to diet and lifestyle, and how to strengthen and heal the body using a range of techniques, incorporating yoga, colour healing, crystals, massage and much more.

What is ayurveda?

Ayurveda is the art of living a balanced life. This is the path to good health, happiness and longevity, and Ayurveda teaches a broad-based doctrine of holistic living with practical instructions on how we may best achieve this.

Rooted in the philosophical and spiritual traditions of India, at the heart of Ayurveda is the understanding that everything in the universe is interconnected: we are not isolated individuals but are part of the greater whole, linked to the web of life by invisible energy pathways, or prana, the "breath of life". Similarly, within each of us, every-thing is connected and operating on many different levels. Ayurveda recognizes that our emotions, intellect and physical body, together with our actions and surrounding environment, are all interlinked and influence each other. Good health is achieved when all these aspects are balanced and in proportion with one another. This leads to inner

▼ CRYSTALS HELP TO CHANNEL ENERGY AS PART OF THE AYRUVEDIC HEALING PROCESS.

▼ IN AYURVEDA MEDITATION HELPS TO BALANCE THE THE BODY, MIND AND SPIRIT.

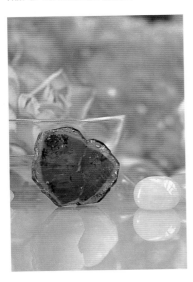

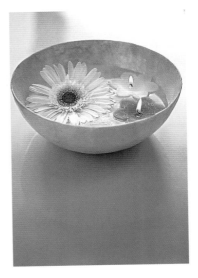

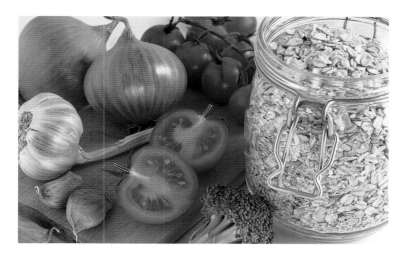

harmony and equilibrium – a feeling of being "at one" with the world and oneself.

There are eight branches to the "tree" of Ayurveda, each one covering various aspects of health and healing, including surgery, gynaecology, paediatrics and medicine. Ayurvedic medicine is the branch responsible for treating our health on a day-to-day basis. Its aim is to prevent and treat ill-health so that we are left free to develop our spiritual potential. This does not mean that you have to have any particular religious belief to benefit from Ayurvedic medicine as the philosophy both acknowledges the uniqueness of the individual, and

▲ CHOOSING A HEALTHY DIET THAT SUITS OUR DOSHA IS THE BASIS OF WELL-BEING.

is also very practical in its applications. It is founded on the belief that all diseases stem from the digestive system and are caused by poor digestion and/or by following an improper diet.

Ayurveda's primary method of treatment is through nutrition, supported by the use of herbs, massage and aromatic oils, but there are also many other outlets, including yoga and meditation, crystals and colour healing. It is about finding what works for you and then applying it to improve your life in whatever ways seem most fitting.

Elemental energies

Everything in the universe is shaped by the cosmic energies of space (or ether), air, fire, water and earth. These forces combine into three fundamental life energies, or doshas, of the human body; vata, pitta and kapha.

The elements are graded beginning with ether, the highest, lightest and most rare, followed by air, then fire and water. The density of earth makes it the heaviest element. Each dosha is a combination of two elements, which predisposes them towards certain principles.

Ayurveda recognizes that each individual is a creation of cosmic energies and a unique phenomenon. No other person has an identical dosha pattern to our own. The combination of vata, pitta and kapha in each of us is determined at conception and is influenced by the season, time of day, and the genetics, diet, lifestyle and emotional state of our parents. Some people are born with a constitution in which all three doshas are equally balanced, which suggests exceptionally good health and a long life span.

However, in most of us, one or two doshas predominate. This unique and specific combination of the doshas is referred to as the "prakruti", our basic nature or constitution. As we experience life's ups

▼ ETHER SUGGESTS A LIGHT AND TRANSIENT STATE. THIS IS THE HIGHEST ELEMENT.

▼ AIR IS HEAVIER THAN ETHER, BUT LIGHTER THAN THE OTHER THREE ELEMENTS.

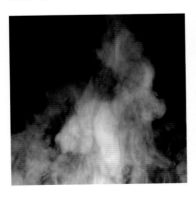

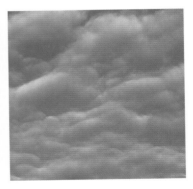

Characteristics of each dosha

dosha	element	cosmic link	character	principle	influence
vata	ether/air	wind	dry/cold	change	activity
pitta	fire/water	sun	hot	conversion	metabolism
kapha	water/earth	moon	moist	inertia	cohesion

and downs, the balance of the doshas in our mind-body system changes. The "vikruti" is our current state of health, influenced by such things as our diet, stress levels, emotional state, physical fitness, and even the weather. If your health is excellent, your vikruti and your prakruti may match. Much more likely, however, is that there will be a discrepancy between the two. The aim of Ayurvedic medicine is to re-establish the balance required by your prakruti.

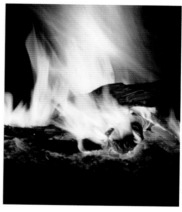

▲ FIRE HAS THE QUALITIES OF HEAT AND DRYNESS. IT IS MIDWAY IN THE ELEMENTS.

▼ WATER SUGGESTS COOL, SMOOTH AND SOFT QUALITIES. IT DESCENDS INTO EARTH.

▼ EARTH IS THE HEAVIEST OF THE FIVE ELEMENTS AND SUGGESTS A SLOW ENERGY.

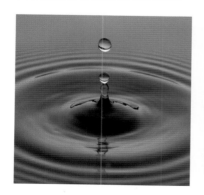

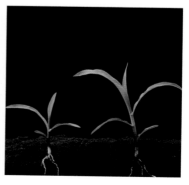

elemental energies **261**

Lifestyle influences

The theory of the doshas is central to Ayurvedic medicine. All bodily, mental and spiritual functions are controlled by the vital forces of vata, pitta and kapha. Health is achieved when these forces are working in harmony.

The subtle energies of vata, pitta and kapha cannot be perceived by any of the senses, yet they are thought to move, increase or diminish, and seem invisibly linked. Changes in the balance of one dosha can have a knock-on effect on the others. In fact the word dosha means "that which tends to go out of balance easily".

Imbalance occurs when we go against our own nature (prakruti) over a long period of time.

A modern Western lifestyle and living in an urban environment seems to make us particularly susceptible. Eating an unhealthy or unsuitable diet puts the body under stress. We suffer pollution in our food, air and water, and even the medicines we take have potentially harmful side-effects. We overload our senses by spending too much time on noisy, polluted city streets, working

▼ TAKE TIME TO RELAX AND ENJOY THE COMPANY OF FRIENDS.

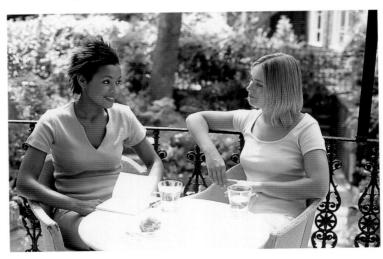

long hours or watching television. There is pressure to live life on the run, eat "fast" food, and overwork in the pursuit of material gain and the realization of goals.

Negative thoughts and emotions affect how we feel, but generally we do not allow ourselves enough time to relax and unwind and to return to mental equilibrium. We tend to forget about the body and its needs and only consider our health when it breaks down and stops us "getting on" with things. When all these factors are taken together, it is hardly surprising that stress-related illnesses are on the increase in the Western world.

However, retreating from life and becoming a hermit is not the answer. Sensory stimulation, desire and challenge are part of life. The approach of Ayurveda is one of balance and it advocates living in tune with nature's laws, paying attention to the rhythms of day and night, the changing seasons and our age. When we get the balance right we live in harmony with our bodies. It is when we go to extremes and pay insufficient attention to the natural patterns of life that we are liable to throw the doshas off balance.

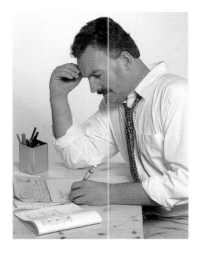

▲ BALANCE YOUR WORKING HOURS WITH RELAXATION, PUTTING THE SAME AMOUNT OF EFFORT INTO EACH.

▼ AYURVEDA TEACHES US TO ATTUNE OUR ATTENTION TO THE NEEDS OF OUR BODIES.

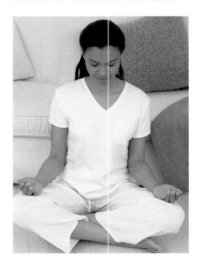

Ayurveda and dis-ease

When the doshas are thrown out of balance their energies become over- or under-stimulated, leading to excess or blocked energy in the body. If these imbalances are left untreated, they will eventually manifest as illness.

The purpose of Ayurveda is to recognize the early warning signs of doshic imbalance so as to "catch" the condition and treat the "dis-ease" before it develops into a serious health problem. If the early warning signs, such as mood swings, low energy levels, persistent aches and pains, or poor digestion over a period of time, are ignored then illness will eventually result.

"Ama"

The main effect of imbalance in the doshas is a build-up of "ama" in the body: these are damaging toxins and waste products. A white coating on the tongue is seen as evidence of ama in the body. The aim of Ayurvedic medicine is to deep-cleanse the system (mind and body) of ama and to restore the balance between the doshas.

▼ Drinking several glasses of water every day helps to flush out toxins.

▼ Massage helps tension to disperse and is pleasant to give and receive.

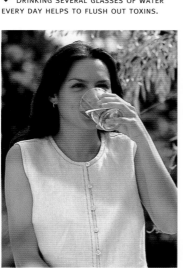

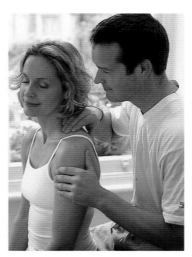

There are many Ayurvedic treatments based on ways to effectively detoxify the system. One simple method is to sip boiled water continuously throughout the day; hot water stimulates the metabolism and encourages the elimination of toxins. Additionally, fasting, eating light meals suitable for your doshic type, meditation and yoga, regular massage and exercise all have a purifying effect on the body and mind. Ayurvedic practitioners advocate moderation in all things to create balance and harmony in the mind and body.

▼ EAT A LIGHT BREAKFAST THAT IS HEALTHY AS WELL AS APPETIZING.

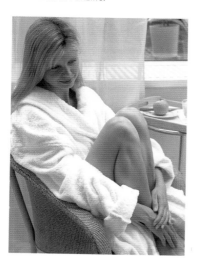

THE SEVEN STAGES TO ILL-HEALTH

Ayurveda sees illness as a gradual process that happens over time and recognizes seven distinct stages. These are states that we are all susceptible to, and some of them are stages that we can actively do something to resolve.

1 Doshic imbalance. This is caused by negative influences, such as poor diet, inadequate rest, environmental pollution or emotional stresses and strains.

2 Aggravation. While the above negative influences continue, the doshas become more seriously unbalanced.

3 Dispersion. The imbalance begins to spread to other parts of the body.

4 Relocation. The affected dosha relocates elsewhere in the body, causing an accumulation of toxic waste products.

5 Mild symptoms. These show in the area where the doshic imbalance is located. It may be at this stage that our attention is brought to our sense of ill-health.

6 Acute illness. In time the symptoms may flare up into an acute condition.

7 Chronic condition. This is the final stage when the symptoms have taken root in the body.

Identifying the doshas

Vata, pitta and kapha are associated with psychological and physical characteristics that influence how we look, think, feel and function. Ayurveda uses these distinctions to determine our constitution (prakruti) and state of health (vikruti).

The characteristics of the doshas are influenced by the elemental energies that make them up. Ayurveda recognizes specific states: there are hot and cold people, thin and fat people, dry and moist people. These body types will have different tendencies emotionally, mentally and physically, and therefore will be affected by different types of food and need different approaches to treatment.

Ayurveda stresses the importance of following the correct diet and lifestyle for your dosha. A basic approach to Ayurveda is to first identify your dosha, at the levels of both prakruti and vikruti and then learn how to eat and live in accordance with this information. If the vikruti is different from the prakruti, you should begin by dealing with the vikruti first, following the guidelines for how to heal your current emotional, physical or mental health conditions with the use of diet and other basic Ayurvedic methods. The aim of treatment is to bring you back to your prakruti, where you can then follow the diet and lifestyle guidelines for your dosha type to maintain balance for lasting health and well-being.

Use the self-assessment chart on the following pages to determine your dosha type. Fill it out twice, using a tick for the prakruti, and a cross for the vikruti. For an objective view, you could also ask someone who knows you well to fill it out for you.

◀ VATA PEOPLE ARE LIGHT IN WEIGHT AND TALL OR VERY SHORT.

To determine your vikruti, concentrate upon your current condition and recent health history. To discover your prakruti, base your choices on what seems most consistently true over your whole lifetime. When you have finished, add up the marks under each dosha to discover your balance in prakruti and vikruti. Most people will have the highest score in one dosha. However, if your score is almost equal between two doshas, then you are probably a dual dosha type, or if equal between three, a tri-dosha type.

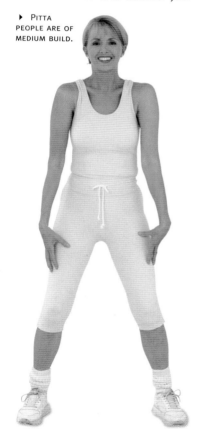

▶ PITTA PEOPLE ARE OF MEDIUM BUILD.

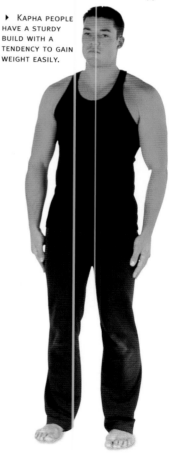

▶ KAPHA PEOPLE HAVE A STURDY BUILD WITH A TENDENCY TO GAIN WEIGHT EASILY.

Which dosha are you?

	VATA	PITTA	KAPHA	V	P	K
Height	Tall or short and thin	Medium	Tall or short and sturdy	☐	☐	☐
Musculature	Thin, prominent tendons	Medium/firm	Plentiful/solid	☐	☐	☐
Bodily frame	Light, narrow	Medium	Large/broad	☐	☐	☐
Weight	Light, hard to gain	Medium	Heavy, gains easily	☐	☐	☐
Sweat	Minimal	Profuse, especially when hot	Moderate	☐	☐	☐
Skin	Dry, cold	Soft, warm	Moist, cool, possibly oily	☐	☐	☐
Complexion	Darkish	Fair/pink/ red/freckles	Pale/white	☐	☐	☐
Hair amount	Average	Early thinning and greying	Plentiful	☐	☐	☐
Type of hair	Dry/thin/ dark/coarse	Fine/soft/ red/fair	Thick, lustrous brown	☐	☐	☐
Size of eyes	Small, narrow or sunken	Average	Large, prominent	☐	☐	☐
Type of eyes	Dark brown or grey, dull	Blue/grey/ hazel, intense	Blue, brown, attractive	☐	☐	☐
Teeth and gums	Protruding, receding gums	Yellowish, gums bleed	White teeth, strong gums	☐	☐	☐
Size of teeth	Small or large, irregular	Average	Large	☐	☐	☐
Physical activity	Quick pace, active	Moderate, average	Slow, steady	☐	☐	☐
Endurance	Low	Good	Very good	☐	☐	☐
Strength	Poor	Good	Very good	☐	☐	☐

	VATA	PITTA	KAPHA	V	P	K
Temperature	Dislikes cold, likes warmth	Likes coolness	Aversion to cool and damp	☐	☐	☐
Digestion	Irregular, forms gas	Quick eating causes burning	Prolonged, forms mucus	☐	☐	☐
Stools	Tendency to constipation	Tendency to loose stools	Plentiful, slow elimination	☐	☐	☐
Lifestyle	Variable, erratic	Busy, tends to achieve a lot	Steady	☐	☐	☐
Sleep	Light, interrupted, fitful	Sound, short	Deep, likes plenty	☐	☐	☐
Emotional tendency	Fearful, anxious, insecure	Fiery, angry, judgemental	Greedy, possessive	☐	☐	☐
Mental activity	Restless, lots of ideas	Sharp, precise, logical	Calm, steady, stable	☐	☐	☐
Memory	Good recent memory	Sharp, generally good	Good long term	☐	☐	☐
Reaction to stress	Excites very easily	Quick temper	Not easily irritated	☐	☐	☐
Work	Creative	Intellectual	Caring	☐	☐	☐
Moods	Change quickly	Change slowly	Generally steady	☐	☐	☐
Speech	Fast	Clear, sharp, precise	Deep, slow	☐	☐	☐
Finances	Poor	Spends on luxuries	Rich, good at saving	☐	☐	☐
Resting pulse:						
Women	Above 80	70–80	Below 70	☐	☐	☐
Men	Above 70	60–70	Below 60	☐	☐	☐
			TOTALS	☐	☐	☐

Vata types

Vata is the energy of movement, and regulates all activity in the body, both mental and physiological, from breathing and blinking to the beating of our hearts. All the impulses in the network of the nervous system are governed by vata.

Vata individuals usually have light, flexible bodies and tend not to gain weight easily. Their tendency is towards dry hair and cool skin and, with little fat to protect them, to feel the cold. Most vata types feel

▼ VATA IS A CREATIVE DOSHA – MANY ARTISTS, DANCERS AND WRITERS ARE VATA TYPES.

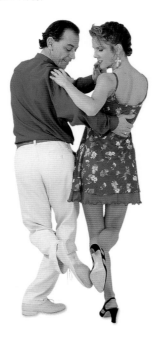

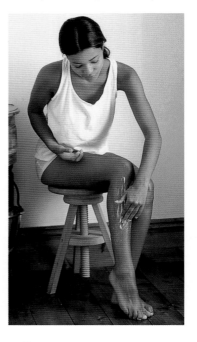

▲ VATA PEOPLE ARE PRONE TO EXCESSIVELY DRY SKIN, CRACKED HEELS AND DRY LIPS.

most comfortable during the spring and summer seasons.

Their constitution is delicate and their levels of energy erratic; they may find it hard to maintain order and structure in their daily lives, quickly becoming bored with routine or mundane tasks. A bundle of nervous energy, the vata type is always on the go, preferring to jog or work out rather than to sit down and take it easy. These individuals may find it hard to relax, which in turn can lead to insomnia and stress-related disorders.

Vata people are clear, quick thinkers, with a highly developed imaginative and intuitive faculty; some may possess clairvoyant abilities. Despite being fearful, anxious types, these people enjoy new challenges and love excitement: they seem to make major life changes, such as change of residence, partner, or employment for instance, much more frequently than other more "grounded" dosha types. This can easily upset their balance and lead to vata disorders.

Balanced vata characteristics

- flexible
- artistic, creative
- imaginative, inventive
- changeable
- fresh, light
- emotions: joy and happiness

Excess vata symptoms

- digestive disorders: constipation, flatulence
- lower back pain, sciatica, arthritis
- nervous disorders
- premenstrual tension
- mental confusion, hyperactivity, restlessness
- emotions: fearful, nervous, anxious, capricious, impatient, irritable

▶ Vata people are prone to dry hair.

Guidelines for balancing vata

- keep warm
- slow down and stay calm
- eat regular meals
- eat cooked, rather than raw food
- spend time alone
- keep a regular routine
- put energy into creative pursuits

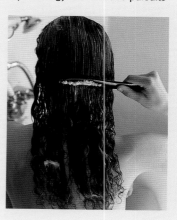

Pitta types

Pitta is the energy of metabolism. It governs all the bio-chemical changes that take place in the body, regulating temperature and digestion, absorption and assimilation – not only of food, but also environmental, external stimuli.

Pittas have a strong constitution; they enjoy their food and have a healthy appetite. Their body type is usually of average build and nicely proportioned, seldom gaining or losing much weight. Generally they have straight, fine, fair hair and skin that is sensitive to the sun. Their eyes are bright and typically blue, greyish-green or coppery brown. Pittas tend to be

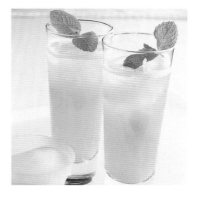

▲ PITTA TYPES MAY NEED TO DRINK MORE IN ORDER TO STAY COOL.

▼ TO BALANCE THEIR WORKAHOLIC NATURE PITTA PEOPLE SHOULD MAKE SURE THEY SPEND TIME IN NATURAL SURROUNDINGS.

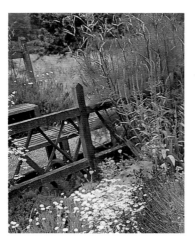

warm and sweat easily, and are aggravated by hot, humid weather.

Pitta types have a keen intellect and a logical, enquiring mind. They love planning and order, and make good leaders and public speakers; they are often attracted to professions such as medicine, engineering and the law, as they enjoy the challenge of going deeply into problems to find a solution. Ambitious, determined and aggressive by nature, their deep-seated fear of failure drives them to succeed. Pitta types are often found reading or working late into the night and many become workaholics, burning their energy through too much mental activity.

Their perfectionist tendencies can make them impatient and intolerant – both towards others and themselves – whereupon they become critical, impatient and judgemental. They are also quick to flare up in anger and are inclined towards jealousy.

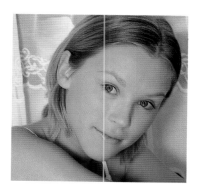

▲ PITTA PEOPLE HAVE A GOOD SENSE OF HUMOUR AND A WARM PERSONALITY.

BALANCED PITTA CHARACTERISTICS

- keen intellect
- meticulous and precise
- capacity for leadership and organization
- enjoys new challenges
- emotions: happiness, humour, warmth

EXCESS PITTA SYMPTOMS

- fevers
- diarrhoea
- inflammatory diseases
- acid indigestion
- skin rashes, eczema
- eye disorders
- premature greying, hair loss
- emotions: anger, hate, irritability, jealousy, envy, fear, bewilderment

▶ PITTA PEOPLE BENEFIT FROM COOLING SHOWERS.

GUIDELINES FOR BALANCING PITTA

- stay cool: cool showers, cool environments, cool drinks
- avoid hot, spicy food
- take time off to relax and slow down
- relax in natural surroundings
- drink more water

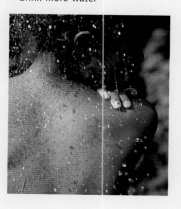

Kapha types

This is the energy of stability, forming the body's structure and supplying the fluids that lubricate the joints, moisturize the skin and heal wounds. It creates and repairs the body's cells, maintains immunity and nourishes our emotions.

The kapha body type is well built, with strong muscles and large, heavy bones. Kapha individuals have thick or fine or wavy hair, smooth skin and large, attractive eyes. They enjoy deep, prolonged sleep and have a steady appetite and thirst, but their slow metabolism and digestion means they have a tendency to gain weight easily, especially if they don't take enough exercise. Although they are naturally athletic and have plenty of stamina, they are not easily motivated into action – a typical kapha type is happy to sit, eat and do nothing. Winter and early spring are the most difficult seasons for a kapha, when the weather is heavy, wet and cold and it is even more difficult to get motivated to keep exercising regularly.

The kapha individual dislikes change and is happiest following a

▼ KAPHA PEOPLE ARE LOVING AND
DEPENDABLE BY NATURE.

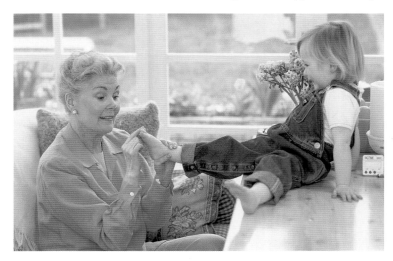

regular routine. They are steady, methodical, practical and pragmatic people – the workers who can be relied upon to get a job done. They have good organizational skills and usually make excellent managers. Additionally, their warm, loving, sensitive nature makes them well suited to the caring professions. Their calm, grounded presence instils confidence in others, acting as a steadying influence on those who are "all over the place".

It is easy for kapha people to get stuck in a rut and fall into lethargy and depression. Once depressed, it becomes even more difficult for them to motivate themselves, and they frequently turn to food for emotional support.

BALANCED KAPHA CHARACTERISTICS

- strength and stamina
- slow and steady
- health and vigour
- good long-term memory
- practical and reliable
- emotions: sweet, loving, sensitive, patient, nurturing

EXCESS KAPHA SYMPTOMS

- congestion
- excess mucus: bronchial/nasal discharge
- sluggish digestion
- slow mental responses
- obesity and fluid retention
- diabetes
- depression
- too much sleep
- emotions: stubbornness, greed, jealousy, possessiveness, lethargy

▶ KAPHA PEOPLE BENEFIT FROM STRONG COLOURS AND REGULAR ACTIVITY.

GUIDELINES FOR BALANCING KAPHA

- wear bright, strong and invigorating colours
- take regular exercise
- avoid heavy, sweet food and dairy products
- vary your routine
- keep active

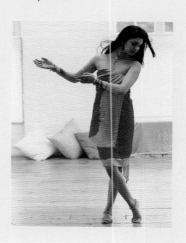

Vata dietary guidelines

Nourishing stews, warming soups and hot, spicy food are good for vata people, whereas cold, raw food is best avoided. To balance their restless nature, they should eat at regular times in a calm, relaxing atmosphere.

HERBS AND SPICES
best source: most of them – particularly warming or sweet herbs; asafoetida helps with the digestion of food.
avoid: caraway.

GRAINS
best source: cooked oats, quinoa, rice, and wheat.
avoid: barley, buckwheat, rye, corn, cereals (cold, dry or puffed), couscous, muesli (granola) and millet.

▼ ALL TYPES OF NUTS AND SEEDS ARE GOOD FOR VATA IF EATEN IN MODERATION.

BEANS, PEAS AND LENTILS
best source: chickpeas, mung beans, red lentils.
avoid: all, except those listed.

MEAT, FISH AND EGGS
best source: beef, chicken, duck, freshwater or sea-fish, shellfish and turkey; boiled or scrambled eggs.
avoid: lamb, pork, rabbit and venison.
• Meat and fish are grounding and strengthening for vata.

▼ ALL FRESH, RIPE FRUITS ARE GOOD FOR THE VATA DIET.

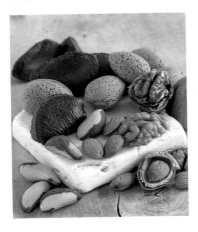

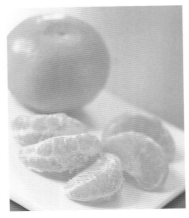

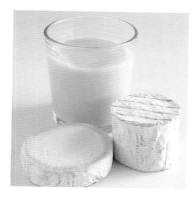

▲ DAIRY PRODUCTS ARE GOOD, ESPECIALLY COW'S AND GOAT'S MILK AND SOFT CHEESE.

VEGETABLES

best source: asparagus, beetroot (beet), carrots, courgettes (zucchini), cucumber, green beans, garlic, leeks, okra, olives, onions (cooked), parsnips, peas, pumpkins, spinach, swede (rutabaga), sweet potatoes and watercress.

avoid: beansprouts, broccoli, Brussels sprouts, cabbage, cauliflower; hot chillies, mushrooms and white potatoes.

• Cooked vegetables are better than those that are raw or dried.

FRUIT

best source: most ripe, sweet fruit.
avoid: cranberries, dried fruit, pears, persimmon, pomegranate, unripe fruit and watermelon.

COOKING OILS

best source: unrefined sesame oil.

SWEETENERS

best source: in moderation: honey, maple syrup and unrefined cane sugar products.
avoid: white sugar.

DRINKS

best source: some fruit juices, beer or wine in moderation, hot dairy drinks, herbal teas, especially chamomile, lavender, licorice, fresh ginger, peppermint and rosehip.
avoid: black tea, coffee, carbonated drinks, ice-cold drinks – tomato, cranberry, pear and apple juice.

▼ HOT CHOCOLATE IS A GOOD CHOICE OF HOT DRINK IF IT IS MADE WITH MILK.

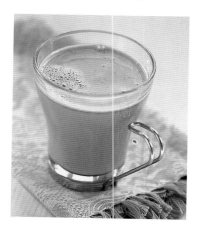

Pitta dietary guidelines

Pitta people should choose cooling and soothing foods, and avoid hot, sour, spicy dishes and fatty, fried or oily food. It is important to eat when hungry, as pitta types easily suffer low blood-sugar levels and become irritable.

HERBS AND SPICES

best source: aloe vera juice (not to be used in pregnancy), basil leaves, cinnamon, coriander (cilantro), cumin, dill, fennel, fresh ginger, hijiki, mint leaves and spearmint.

avoid: all hot spices, cayenne and chilli peppers, garlic, salt, vinegar, mustard seeds and ketchup.

GRAINS

best source: barley, oats, wheat, and rice (especially white basmati).

avoid: brown rice, buckwheat, corn, millet and rye.

▼ CINNAMON IS A MILD, VERSATILE SPICE THAT IS A GOOD CHOICE FOR PITTA PEOPLE.

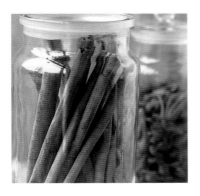

BEANS, PEAS AND LENTILS

best source: all beans, chickpeas, tofu and other unfermented soya products.

avoid: green lentils (except in soup) and red lentils; miso, soy sauce.

NUTS AND SEEDS

best source: almonds, coconut, pumpkin and sunflower seeds.

avoid: all others, particularly cashew nuts and sesame seeds.

MEAT, FISH AND EGGS

best source: in strict moderation: chicken, freshwater fish, rabbit, turkey and venison.

avoid: red meat, all seafood and egg yolk.

VEGETABLES

best source: most, especially asparagus, broccoli, green leaf vegetables, green lettuce, chicory.

avoid: carrots, aubergines (eggplant), spinach, radishes, onions, raw beetroot (beet), green olives, peppers, kohlrabi and tomatoes.

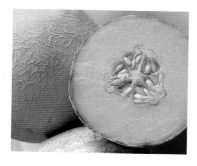

▲ SWEET RIPE MELON IS BENEFICIAL FOR PITTA PEOPLE.

• Include plenty of salads and raw, rather than cooked vegetables in your diet.

FRUIT
best source: fully ripe, sweet, fresh fruit, including apples, apricots, avocados, berries, cherries, dates, figs, mangoes, melons, papaya, pears and plums.
avoid: citrus fruits, fruits with a sour or sharp, tangy taste such as cranberries, rhubarb, strawberries and green grapes.

DAIRY PRODUCTS
best source: most in moderation.
avoid: salted butter, buttermilk, sour cream and yogurt.

COOKING OILS
best source: in moderation: olive, sunflower, soya, coconut and walnut oils.
avoid: almond, corn and sesame oils.

SWEETENERS
best source: most in moderation.
avoid: honey and molasses.

DRINKS
best source: most sweet fruit juices, cow's milk, soya milk, rice milk mixed vegetable juice, beer and black tea.
avoid: hard spirits, wine, caffeinated drinks, sour or sharp fruit juices (such as berry juices), tomato juice and any ice-cold drinks.

▼ PITTA PEOPLE SHOULD EAT HARD CHEESES SUCH AS CHEDDAR IN MODERATION.

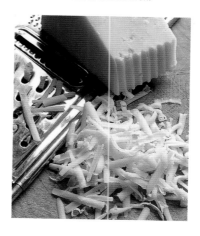

Kapha dietary guidelines

Kapha food should be light, dry, hot and stimulating. Opt for cooked foods in preference to salads but go easy on rich sauces. Dairy products, sweet, sour and salty tastes and an excessive intake of wheat all aggravate kapha.

HERBS AND SPICES
best source: all pungent spices – ginger, black pepper, coriander (cilantro), turmeric and cardamom.
avoid: salt.

GRAINS
best source: barley, buckwheat, corn, couscous, millet, oat bran, polenta, rye.
avoid: oat flakes, pasta, wheat and rice (brown and white).

▾ MOST BEANS ARE GOOD FOR THE KAPHA DIET.

NUTS AND SEEDS
best source: pumpkin and sunflower seeds.
avoid: all nuts.

BEANS, PEAS AND LENTILS
avoid: kidney beans, soy beans (and their products), tofu (cold) and miso.

MEAT, FISH AND EGGS
best source: in strict moderation:

▾ FRESHWATER FISH IS BETTER THAN SEAWATER FISH FOR KAPHAS.

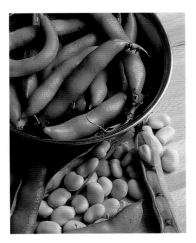

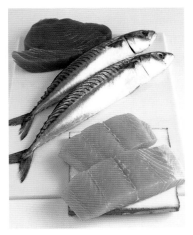

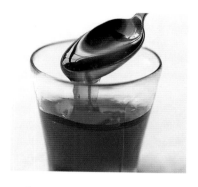

▲ HONEY IS THE BEST SWEETENER, BUT YOU SHOULD AVOID SUGAR AND MOLASSES.

scrambled eggs, poultry, prawns (shrimp), rabbit and venison.
avoid: beef, lamb, pork, seafood (except prawns/shrimp).

VEGETABLES
best source: most.
avoid: sweet vegetables, such as courgettes (zucchini), cucumber, parsnips, sweet potatoes, pumpkin, squash and tomatoes.
• Cooked vegetables are best.

FRUIT
best source: apples, apricots, berries, cherries, cranberries, peaches, pears, pomegranates, prunes and raisins.
avoid: bananas, kiwi fruits, avocados, coconuts, dates, melons, olives, papaya, plums and pineapple.

• Sharp, astringent fruits are better than sweet or sour ones.

COOKING OILS
best source: corn, almond or sunflower oil.
• Use fats and oils sparingly.

DRINKS
best source: fresh fruit and vegetable juices, black tea, herbal teas, hot soy milk drinks, dry red or white wine very occasionally.
avoid: fizzy, caffeinated drinks, coffee, orange juice, tomato juice and iced drinks.

▼ SQUASH IS A SWEET-TASTING VEGETABLE AND SHOULD BE AVOIDED BY KAPHA PEOPLE. SWEET FOODS HINDER A KAPHA'S ENERGY.

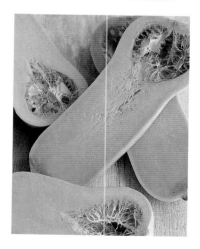

Optimum living

Ayurveda stresses the importance of living a balanced life. It is all very well following the dietary guidelines for our dosha type, but if we neglect to take care of ourselves in the rest of our lives, then our efforts will be less effective.

Regular exercise plays an important role in staying healthy for all dosha types. It keeps the body strong and stimulates the digestive system to work more effectively.

Kaphas will get the most benefit from vigorous exercise, such as running, fast swimming, aerobics and fitness training, which will help to cleanse the body and dispel sluggish, lazy feelings. Kaphas should exercise more when the weather is cold and damp. Pittas require a moderate amount of

▼ THE TYPE OF EXERCISE YOU SHOULD DO IS DETERMINED BY YOUR CONSTITUTION.

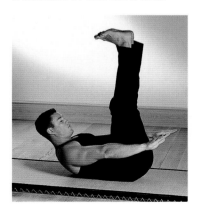

exercise, done for the fun of it rather than to be top dog; jogging, team sports and tai chi are all good. Vata people benefit from gentle, relaxing forms of exercise. They are the most easily exhausted of the dosha types, so they should not overdo things. Walking, yoga and slow swimming are ideal, although vata people can undertake most sports and activities, so long as they don't push themselves beyond their limits.

ROUTINE

Keeping a regular routine for vital activities such as sleeping, eating, exercising, bathing and working helps us to maintain balance in our lives. Ayurveda recommends harmonizing our internal body clock with the natural rhythm of the day. Long-distance travel, working night shifts, and eating at irregular times can all throw our body clock, and the doshas, off balance, making us feel out of sorts and out of harmony with those around us.

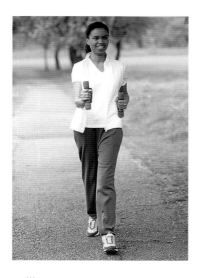

▲ WE ARE AT OUR MOST ACTIVE BETWEEN 10AM AND 2PM.

THE DAILY CYCLE

Ayurveda divides the day into two cycles, which roughly correspond with day and night. Each cycle has three phases, governed by one of the doshas.

DAY

06.00–10.00 kapha time of day. The body is gathering energy to begin the day. This is the best time for purification rituals (shower, cleansing, eliminating), yoga and meditation. Eat a light breakfast.

10.00–14.00 pitta time of day. The appetite is strongest at lunch-time so have your main meal of the day between these hours.

14.00–18.00 vata time of day. This is the most creative and communicative time of the day. Take a regular break to avoid activity turning into stress. The late afternoon is a good time to meditate.

NIGHT

18.00–22.00 kapha time of night. The body tires. Eat a light meal and take a walk to aid digestion.

22.00–02.00 pitta time of night. Avoid strenuous activity. Go to bed at a reasonable hour.

02.00–06.00 vata time of night. The body shuts down.

▼ ALL DOSHAS SHOULD ADOPT A ROUTINE THAT ADHERES TO THE NATURAL RHYTHM OF THE DAY AND NIGHT.

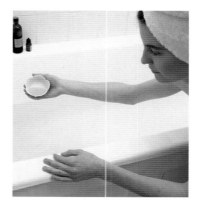

The cycles of life

The seasons of the year show us that life is cyclical; an ever-lasting round of gestation, birth, growth, decline and death. The doshas are inevitably related to these natural laws and follow this regenerative cycle.

The doshas are sensitive to changes in weather conditions, which loosely tie in with the seasons. Vata is highest in autumn and early winter, and at times of dry, cold and windy weather. The pitta season is late spring and summer and during times of heat and humidity. Kapha is highest in the winter months and during early spring when the weather is cold and damp.

Ayurveda recommends that we take these seasonal changes into account when we are planning our eating and lifestyle habits, as the weather can aggravate or cause doshic imbalance. For instance, during the cold, damp months of winter, kapha accumulates. This leads to more "damp" in the body in the form of excess mucus, and is the traditional season for coughs and colds. This is made much more likely if your diet is high in foods that aggravate the kapha condition – lots of dairy products and heavy, rich food – and more likely still if

▼ SPRING IS THE TIME TO CONSIDER A CLEANSING FAST TO CLEAR EXCESS KAPHA.

▼ SUMMER IS THE SEASON OF HEAT. COUNTER IT WITH SOOTHING ACTIVITIES.

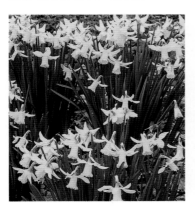

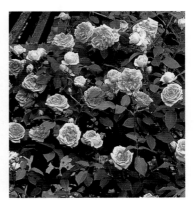

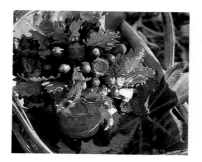

▲ Autumn is the season of changeable
weather and increased levels of vata.

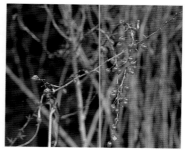

▲ Kapha people find it hard to motivate
themselves in winter.

you are a kapha or have a kapha imbalance (vikruti).

If you are a dual or tri-dosha type, work with whichever dosha predominates at any given time. For example, if you are a vata-pitta type, choose foods from the pitta eating plan during the summer months and from the vata plan during the autumn and winter.

The stages of life

Ayurveda also sees the human life span in terms of the doshas.

0–30 years – kapha: this is the time of growth and development.

30–60 years – pitta: we apply the skills and knowledge of our kapha years to this time of life.

60+ years – vata: physical decline and spiritual growth.

WEATHER/SEASON	VATA	PITTA	KAPHA	BEST ACTION
warming up (spring)	neutral	accumulating	aggravated	cleansing fast to clear excess kapha
hot (summer)	accumulating	aggravated	decreasing	wear cooling colours, eat raw foods, rest and relax
cooling (autumn)	aggravated	decreasing	neutral	stay warm and comfortable; follow a regular routine
cold (winter)	decreasing	neutral	accumulating	treat kapha dosha with spices and warm drinks

Yoga

An important element of Ayurvedic therapy is yoga as an exercise and a therapy. It is not only a physical discipline that helps to keep the body strong and supple, but it also calms the mind and helps us to find inner peace.

Yoga works with a variety of techniques, including physical postures, breathing exercises, relaxation and meditation. In its purest form it is a preparation for spiritual enlightenment, but it is also an effective therapy in the treatment of stress and chronic disease conditions.

Vata types are particularly suited to the gentle, rhythmic nature of yoga exercise, but all three doshas can benefit from yoga.

STANDING WARM-UPS

Before practising yoga, it is best to warm-up and stretch out the body. Stand relaxed but tall with the spine erect and the feet hip-width apart. Bring your hands together in front of your chest into prayer position. Raise your arms to the sides and come up on to your toes. Breathe in and stretch the arms up. Then breathe out to lower the arms and heels. Get a vigorous swinging movement going, opening the chest, stretching the spine and "waking up" the circulation.

SALUTE TO THE SUN

The following routine is best practised on rising first thing in the morning. The sequence should be repeated between two and six times. It is a good exercise to get yourself moving and release sluggish, tired feelings.

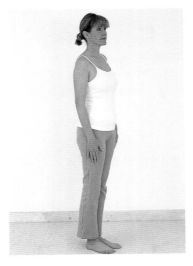

1 Stand upright with your hands at your side, knees and shoulders relaxed and your neck fully extended upwards. Inhale.

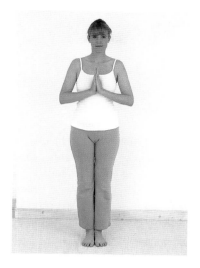

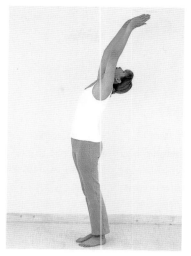

2 Look straight ahead. Breathe out while bringing the palms of your hands together at chest height into the prayer position.

3 Breathe in deeply. Keeping your hands together, raise your hands over your head. Arch your back as far as is comfortable. Exhale slowly.

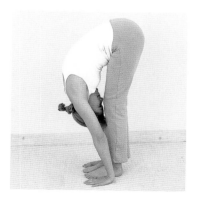

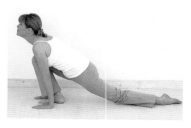

4 Bend forward to touch the floor if you can, at each side of your feet.

5 Breathing in, bend your right knee and slide and extend your left leg out behind you. Your knee rests on the floor. Put the hands on the floor. Extend your neck upwards.

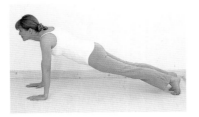

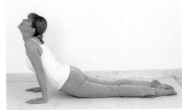

6 With your hands flat on the floor, extend your right leg out to meet your left leg. Take your weight up on to your hands and your toes. Keep the neck straight. Breathe out. Lower the body flat to the ground.

7 Supporting the weight of your upper body on your arms, raise your chest, stomach and pelvic bones from the ground. Extend your neck upwards. Exhale slowly. Breathing in, lower your stomach and pelvis back down to the floor.

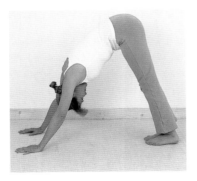

8 In one movement, raise your bottom and pull yourself up into an arch. Extend your arms and legs fully. Lower your heels towards the floor (but don't strain). Bend your left knee so that it touches the ground part way between your right foot and hands. Bring the right foot to the side of the left knee.

TYPES OF YOGA

There are many different types of yoga. The most widely practised in the West is "Hatha" yoga. Hatha yoga is just one branch of yoga and within this branch there are various sub-categories.

• Astanga Vinyasa: a fast series of challenging postures performed using synchronized breathing. This is probably the most aerobic form of yoga.

• Iyengar: alignment and precision of movement are used to enhance posture, breathing and flexibility.

• Kundalini: breathing techniques and prana (life force) are worked on to balance the body's energy and achieve relaxation.

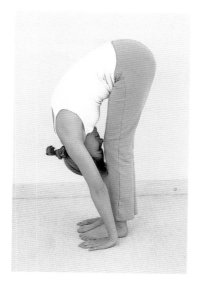

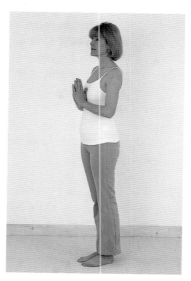

9 Move your hands back to your feet and return to position 4

10 Breathe in deeply as you raise your torso and repeat step 2.

11 Breathe out slowly as you lower your arms and return to the starting position. Look straight ahead, allow your breathing to return to normal, then repeat the whole sequence with the other leg.

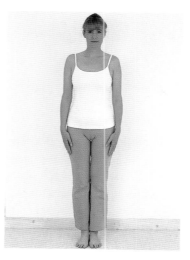

CAUTION

This sequence is not suitable during pregnancy, during the menstrual cycle, or if you are suffering from any physical injury or back pain.

Body shaping

A sensuous shape relies on well-toned muscles. That means some kind of strength-building work, but adding some stretches is vital if you want to firm up without adding bulk. The stretching element is built into yoga.

THE CAT (CHAKRAVAKASANA)

This tones muscles in the back, arms and buttocks and stretches the hamstrings.

1 Kneel on all fours with shoulders above wrists, hips above knees and soles turned up. As you breathe in, arch your back downwards so that your waist sinks lower than your hips and shoulders. Lift your head while keeping the neck long.

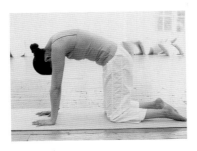

2 As you breathe out, come back to a central position. Continuing the outbreath, arch your back upwards and tuck your chin in towards your chest. Breathe in as you return to the central position. Repeat this movement slowly several times.

THE COBRA (BHUJANGASANA)

This tones buttock muscles and pectorals. Don't risk damaging your neck by tipping your head too far back – keep the neck long.

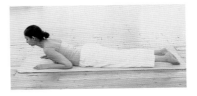

1 Lie on your stomach with your legs stretched out and arms by your sides, palms facing down. Bend your arms and bring your hands beside your shoulders. As you breathe in, slowly raise your chest.

2 On an outbreath, push your palms down and raise your upper body as far as possible while keeping your pubic bone in contact with the floor. As you breathe in again, raise your head slightly. Relax the muscles in your back and buttocks, and feel your spine lengthen. Lower your body to the starting position.

The Bridge (Setu Bandha)

In this pose, you're working on your hips and thighs.

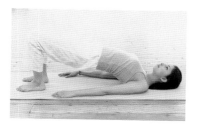

1 Lie on your back, arms by your sides with palms facing downwards. Bring your heels towards your torso, hip-width apart. As you breathe in, raise your buttocks as high as possible, pushing upwards with your pelvis till you are resting on your feet and shoulders. Tuck your chin in and let your head rest on the floor.

2 If this is very easy, try an advanced version. Proceed to the position at the end of step 1, then, keeping your upper arms on the floor, bend your elbows and, as you breathe out, put your hands under your waist for support. Do not flop down on to your hands or push your spine up too high. If it's hard to keep your back raised, come down gently.

Lying-down Twist (Jathara Parivartanasana)

This works on trimming the waist while releasing tension from muscles in the back.

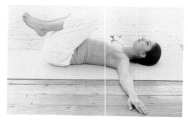

1 Lie on the floor with arms outstretched and palms facing down. Bend your knees and raise them slowly to your chest. Keep your neck and spine in a straight line.

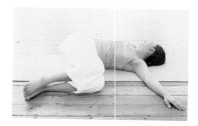

2 On an outbreath, lower your knees to the floor on one side and turn your head to the other. Hold for as long as is comfortable, then slowly come back to the centre on an outbreath, pause for a moment and repeat on the other side.

Relaxing meditation

Meditation is food for the soul. Its effect is to deep-clean the mind and transform the emotions, leaving us feeling refreshed and calm. It is one of the most important methods in Ayurveda for permanently stabilizing the doshas.

Ayurvedic practitioners believe that toxins (ama) in the body also have their emotional and mental counterparts. Emotional states, such as greed, envy, jealousy and anger, negative thoughts and compulsive behaviour patterns create psychic "dirt" or emotional ama. They are as detrimental to our health as the chemical stress hormones produced by the body.

DAILY MEDITATION

Make meditation a part of your daily routine. Practise it for 10–15 minutes a day. Sunrise and sunset are the best times to meditate, but find a time that is convenient for you and stick to it. Some people like to use a (gentle) alarm to indicate when the session is finished.

1 Find a quiet place where you won't be disturbed. Either sit on a straight-backed chair or cross-legged on the floor. It is important that you are relaxed and comfortable and that your spine is straight.

2 Place your hands, palms upmost, on your thighs. Alternatively, rest your hands on your knees or on a small cushion on your lap.

3 Close your eyes and become aware of your breathing. With every out-breath, think "letting go".

4 Focus your attention inwards, allowing any noises or distractions outside to fade away.

▼ THE CLASSIC YOGA POSE, THE LOTUS POSITION, HAS BECOME SYMBOLIC OF RELAXATION AND MEDITATION. HOWEVER, IT TAKES SUPPLE JOINTS AND PRACTISE TO ACHIEVE IT.

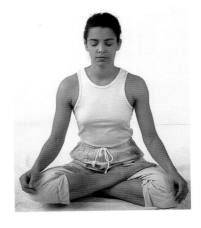

5 Don't try to control your mind – either by trying to hold on to a particular thought, or by rejecting any other. Meditation is all about accepting what you find and just allowing it to be there. Let your mind wander freely.

6 Remember to stay focused on your breath (this will naturally help to quieten the mind) and keep your body relaxed.

7 When you are ready, open your eyes and let yourself return to normal waking consciousness. Slowly get up and have a good stretch, ready to face the world again with renewed vigour.

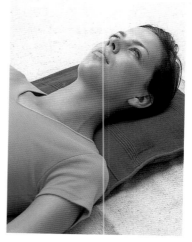

▲ YOU CAN MEDITATE LYING DOWN, BUT DON'T CHOOSE A BED FOR YOUR SURFACE OR YOU MAY FIND YOURSELF FALLING ASLEEP.

▼ AT THE END OF YOUR MEDITATION, HUG YOUR KNEES INTO YOUR CHEST, THEN STRETCH OUT YOUR LIMBS.

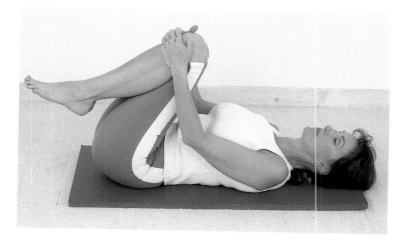

The radiance of colour

Colour is a delight to our visual sense and its subtle vibrations affect us on all levels of our being. Ayurvedic treatments make use of the healing powers of colour to restore or stabilize the balance between the three doshas.

COLOURS AND THE DOSHAS

We can use colour to influence our well-being in the clothes we wear, the food we eat, and in our environment. The vibrations of certain colours help or aggravate each of the doshas.

VATA

Energetic vata individuals benefit from most of the pastel colours and earthy colours that are gentle and warm to look at, such as ochres, browns and yellows. Brown and ochre help to draw energy down through the body's system, stabilizing and grounding the vata personality; yellow is linked to the mind and will help to keep the vata mentally alert. Minimize the use of dark and cool colours, such as blues, browns and black.

PITTA

Excess pitta (such as irritability and impatience) is balanced by wearing cooling and calming colours, such as green, blue, violet, or any quiet pastel shade. Blue is a healing colour and helps the pitta type to remain open without being over-stimulated; green soothes the emotions and encourages harmonious feelings; and violet increases awareness of spiritual issues. Reds and oranges can inflame the pitta dosha, and yellow, gold and black should be minimized.

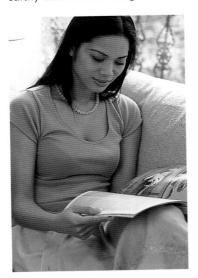

◀ PASTEL COLOURS ARE LIBERATING FOR VATA PEOPLE.

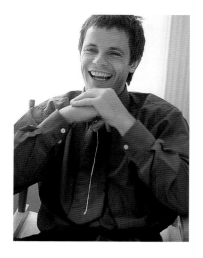

KAPHA

The lethargy of kapha is balanced by bright, lively, bold colours, especially reds, oranges and warm pinks. Both reds and pinks are energizing and positive but red should be used sparingly as it may be over-stimulating. Orange is a warming, nourishing colour that feeds the sexual organs and helps to remove congestion in the system. Yellow and gold are also good colours for kapha, but greens, dark blues or white are best avoided.

▼ KAPHA PEOPLE SHOULD CHOOSE VIBRANT COLOURS TO HELP MOTIVATE THEMSELVES INTO ACTION.

COLOUR INFUSIONS

In Ayurveda colour is an important healing tool. Different colours carry specific energies. To make a colour infusion wrap a piece of coloured fabric or film around a glass of water and leave it to stand in the sun for 4 hours. The water will become infused with the vibrations of that colour, and drinking it is said to bring beneficial results.

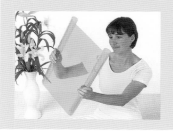

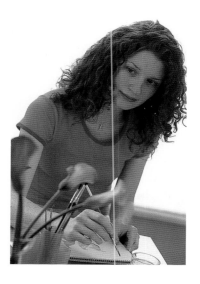

Crystals and gems

All substances in nature are believed to contain the creative intelligence of the cosmos. Gems and crystals have healing energies that enliven the vital energy centres (chakras) in the body, and can be utilized to harmonize the doshas.

Stones are able to act as energy transmitters, having the power to store, magnify and transform energy. This means it is important to always clean any stone before it is used for healing purposes; leave it to soak in salt water overnight and then rinse thoroughly. Once the stone is free from any psychic "dirt", you can then make an infusion by placing it in a glass bowl of spring water and leaving it in sunlight for about 4 hours. Drain off the water and drink it.

VATA

Rose quartz balances excess vata and brings relief to conditions such as nervousness, dry skin and hair, constipation and bloating. Topaz is a warm stone that dispels fear and is ideal for calming vata anxiety; wear it when you want to feel confident and in control. Amethyst has balancing properties and is useful for troublesome emotional states or when clarity of mind is needed.

▼ CRYSTALS ARE IMPORTANT HEALING TOOLS IN AYURVEDA.

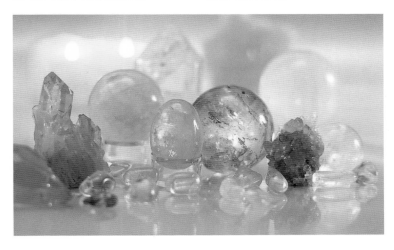

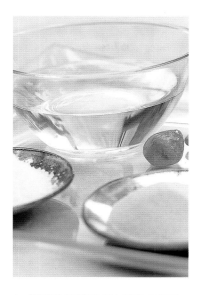

▲ CLEANSE CRYSTALS IN A BOWL OF SALT WATER BEFORE USE.

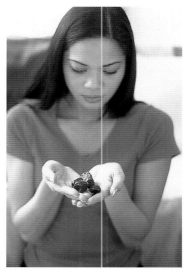

▲ ATTUNE YOUR ATTENTION TO CRYSTALS TO BENEFIT FROM THEIR ENERGY.

It also helps to promote feelings of inner peace and harmony. Quartz crystal also helps to calm vata and enhances intuition.

PITTA

Pearls (or mother-of-pearl), red coral and moonstone are all good for reducing excess pitta. All three stones have a soft and cooling energy vibration that can help to calm inflammatory conditions, such as angry emotions, skin rashes, all "-itises", and acid indigestion. Amethyst encourages compassion and dignity and is also good for pitta imbalances.

KAPHA

Deep red stones, such as ruby or garnet, stimulate kapha energy and balance the effects of excess kapha conditions, including water retention, lethargy, depression, weight problems and sinus and respiratory disorders. The refined, subtle vibrations of lapis lazuli will also help to lift excess kapha from its slow, heavy nature to something more light and ethereal.

Aromas and massage

Our sense of smell is directly related to the balance of the doshas. Fragrant essential oils, extracted from hundreds of different plants and their components, can be used to balance the mind and heal the emotions.

Essential oils are inhaled and/or massaged into the skin. They should not be put directly on the skin or taken internally; some oils are contra-indicated in pregnancy or for some medical conditions.

AROMAS AND THE DOSHAS

Warm, sweet, calming and earthy aromas balance vata. These include camphor, eucalyptus, ginger, musk, sandalwood and jatamansi (a spikenard species from India). A blend of basil, orange, geranium, and cloves is good for harmonizing vata imbalance, and other useful fragrances include lavender, pine and frankincense.

Pitta is soothed by cooling, calming, sweet aromas such as honeysuckle, jasmine, sandalwood and rose. Rose geranium, lemongrass, fennel or mint are helpful.

Warm and stimulating or spicy, earthy fragrances are helpful for kapha. These include eucalyptus, cinnamon, myrrh, thyme, basil, musk, camphor, cloves, rosemary, ginger and sage. Juniper oil is especially useful for lymphatic drainage.

▼ LOOKING AT A ROSE AS WELL AS SMELLING ONE LIFTS THE SPIRITS AND PROMOTES FEELINGS OF WELL-BEING.

▼ ESSENTIAL OILS ARE APPLIED TO THE SKIN IN A "CARRIER" OIL, SUCH AS ALMOND OR WHEATGERM.

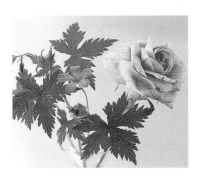

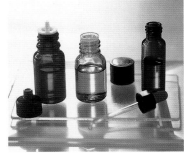

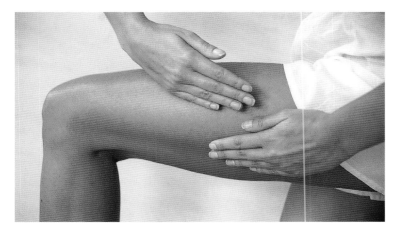

MASSAGE AND THE DOSHAS

To massage with essential oils, add 7–10 drops of the chosen essential oil to 25ml/1½ tbsp carrier oil.

Vatas enjoy gentle, soothing and relaxing massage. Use stroking movements and pay attention to areas of tight, dry skin. Pitta massage should be calming and relaxing. Use deep and varied movements and go easy wherever there is stiffness or soreness.

A vigorous massage stimulates the sluggish kapha metabolism. Use fast and strong movements, using very little oil or none at all (talcum powder may be used instead). To encourage lymphatic drainage, pay particular attention to the hip and groin area and around the armpits.

▲ PITTAS SHOULD HAVE A SLOW MASSAGE RHYTHM AND AVOID SUDDEN MOVEMENTS.

▼ A DAILY FOOT AND HAND MASSAGE WILL ACT AS A GROUNDING AND STABILIZING INFLUENCE FOR VATAS.

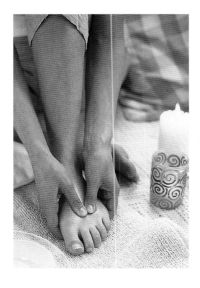

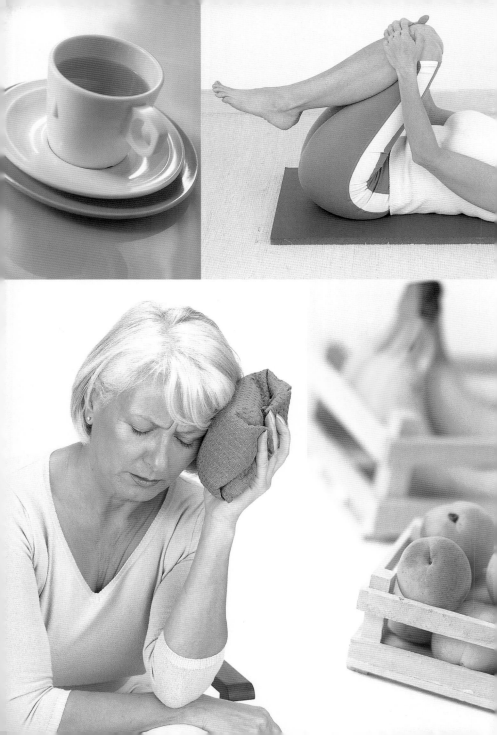

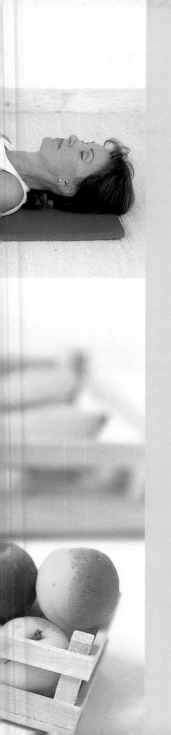

AYURVEDA

FOR COMMON AILMENTS

In Ayurveda, health problems are treated according to dosha. Some conditions may affect vata, pitta or kapha types, while others may be linked to one dosha. Diarrhoea, for example, is a pitta condition, while constipation is a vata one. When treating an ailment, you will need to determine the character of the symptoms, and follow the eating and lifestyle plan for that dosha to bring it back into balance.

Some of treatments in the following section recommend special Ayurvedic herbal remedies. These herbs are available from Ayurvedic Health suppliers and can be obtained via the internet. Always consult a qualified Ayurvedic or medical doctor if your symptoms fail to improve, or if you are unsure.

Digestive disorders

The gastro-intestinal tract is the most important part of the body, and the seat of the doshas. Our dosha type and lifestyle factors all influence the digestive system and each dosha is subject to particular disorders.

Regular bowel movements are a sign of a healthy gastro-intestinal tract (GI). Vata types are prone to irregular digestion and typical vata conditions include constipation, gas/flatulence, and tension (causing stomach cramps or spasms).

CONSTIPATION
Drinking a glass of hot water each morning will help to get things moving. Herbs include triphala and satisabgol (psyllium husks). Triphala is a special Ayurvedic combination of three herbal fruits. It should not

▼ BUY AYURVEDIC HERBS FROM A SPECIALIST STOCKIST.

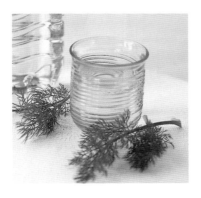

be used during pregnancy or if you suffer from ulcers of the GI. Satisabgol is gentle and soothing and a good "bulking" agent.

GAS, BLOATING AND COLIC
If undigested food stays in the system for too long it begins to ferment, causing a range of unpleasant symptoms. Ayurvedic medicine recommends hingvastak, a herbal mix that includes asafoetida, ginger, black pepper and cumin.

Pitta digestion tends to be too fast. These types easily "burn" up food in anger or frustration and typical pitta problems include acidity and heartburn and diarrhoea.

ACIDITY AND HEARTBURN
Sip aloe vera juice to cool an inflamed digestive system (but not if you are pregnant). Use herbal preparations of shatavari, licorice (not to be used with high blood pressure or oedema) and amalki to balance acidity.

DIARRHOEA

Avoid hot spices and eat small meals. Drink nettle tea to balance the digestive system and add coriander (cilantro), saffron, fresh ginger and nutmeg to your diet. A simple diet of rice, split mung dhal and vegetables is recommended while symptoms last.

The kapha metabolism is slow and problems of the GI lead to obesity, nausea, a build-up of mucus and poor circulation. Herbs for kapha conditions include trikatu ("three hot things"), which contains ginger, pippali and black pepper. Hot spices in general, such as chilli peppers, garlic and ginger are helpful for invigorating and cleansing the system. Regular vigorous exercise will help to keep kapha people moving and avoid stagnation.

◄ IF YOU HAVE A STOMACH UPSET, TRY TAKING A TONIC OF NETTLE TEA. IT WILL HELP TO BALANCE THE DIGESTIVE SYSTEM AND ALLEVIATE PITTA CONDITIONS.

▼ HERBAL TEAS ARE POWERFUL TONICS THAT ARE USED IN AYURVEDA.

▼ CHILLIES ARE GOOD FOR THE KAPHA DIET: THE HEAT OFFSETS THE SLUGGISH NATURE.

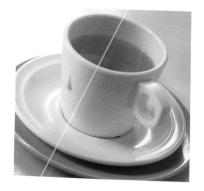

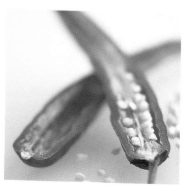

High blood pressure

Hypertension or high blood pressure is a potentially life-threatening condition and must be treated by a qualified medical practitioner. Ayurveda recommends steps that you can take which can help to bring it under control.

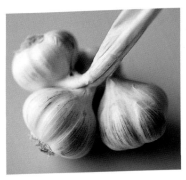

▲ EAT PLENTY OF GARLIC (RAW, FRESH IS BEST) AND TAKE REGULAR EXERCISE.

Lifestyle and diet play an important role in the prevention and treatment of hypertension. Physical and emotional stress cause the blood vessels to constrict and blood pressure to rise. Regular meditation and gentle yoga will help to counter this. A profound and simple way to relax is to lie in corpse pose for 10–15 minutes a day. Inverted postures (such as a headstand or a shoulderstand) and forward bending movements should be avoided.

Hypertension is often linked with high levels of cholesterol – increased lipids (fats) in the blood

and fatty deposits on the artery walls, causing them to narrow. Stick to a kapha-reducing diet: avoiding dairy foods, especially hard cheeses, full-fat milk and sweet foods, salt, fried or cold food, cold drinks and red meat.

HONEY WATER

Add 5ml/1 tsp honey and 5–10 drops of apple cider vinegar or lime juice to a cup of hot water and drink a cup each morning. This helps to "scrape" fat from the system and lower cholesterol levels.

▼ LIMES ARE ACIDIC IN NATURE AND CAN HELP TO REDUCE CHOLESTEROL.

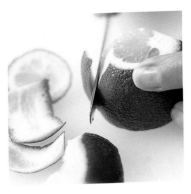

Emotional stress

Our health is a complex interplay between our mind and emotions and our physical body. Mental and emotional stress can lead to physical ill-health and vice versa. Each of the doshas is prone to particular negative emotional states.

VATA

Of all the doshas, vata is the most prone to suffer the effects of stress. Anxiety, fear, insecurity, nervousness, restlessness and confusion are associated with increased vata. Slow down, eat regular, healthy meals and meditate each day. Fresh ginger and lemon tea are good tonics. A lavender, chamomile or jasmine oil massage is calming.

PITTA

Anger, criticism, irritability, frustration, envy and hostility are all signs of aggravated pitta. To cool the temper eat plain foods and cool drinks; avoid tea, coffee and alcohol. Focus on your emotions when you meditate. Include the following herbs in your diet: chamomile, coriander (cilantro), cumin, fennel, tulsi and sandalwood.

KAPHA

Boredom and a "can't be bothered" feeling are signs of unbalanced kapha. This dosha is associated with greed, possessiveness and attachment, which leads to over-eating and to be "greedy" and smothering in relationships. Work with the kapha eating plan, and be sure to take plenty of vigorous exercise. Give the other more "space" in your relationships.

▼ A SOOTHING MASSAGE WON'T TAKE AWAY THE CAUSE OF YOUR EMOTIONAL STRESS BUT WILL HELP TO RELAX YOUR MIND AND BODY.

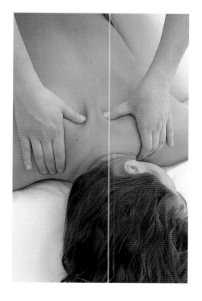

Premenstrual syndrome

Every month, many women experience unpleasant physical and emotional symptoms 7–10 days before their period. For some it is severely debilitating. Ayurveda classifies the symptoms of PMS according to dosha type.

Lower-back pain, lower abdominal pain and bloating, coupled with anxiety, fearfulness, insomnia and marked mood swings are associated with vata imbalance. Take 15ml/1 tbsp aloe vera gel mixed with a pinch of black pepper three times a day before meals. Include the following herbs in your diet: dashamula, kaishore guggulu or yogaraj guggulu.

Pitta-type symptoms include irritability, tender breasts, hives, raised body temperature (hot flushes, sweats) and cystitis. Make a herbal mix of two parts shatavari to one part each of brahmi and musta. Take 2.5ml/½ tsp with warm water, twice a day. Alternatively, add a pinch of cumin powder to 15ml/1 tbsp aloe vera gel and take three times daily.

One of the main features of kapha premenstrual syndrome (PMS) is water retention; the breasts become heavy and swollen, and the legs, feet and ankles may also swell. Emotionally, the woman feels weepy, depressed and lethargic. Add a pinch of trikatu to 15ml/1 tbsp of aloe vera gel and take three times daily. Other herbs to include in your diet are purnarnava, kutki and musta.

◄ FOR MANY WOMEN PMS CAN BE DIFFICULT AND DEBILITATING. MAKE A RECORD OF YOUR SYMPTOMS AND DO NOT IGNORE THEM.

TREATMENT TIPS
To treat vata and kapha PMS, eat ten cherries a day on an empty stomach a week or so before the period starts.

Low libido

Ayurveda acknowledges the importance of a healthy, fulfilling sex life. Our sex drive is affected by high stress levels, emotional factors and also by weakness or debility in the male or female reproductive organs.

Ayurveda suggests many foods that can strengthen the reproductive system. The following are equally suitable for both sexes.

ALMONDS

Soak ten almonds overnight. Peel them and eat before breakfast each day. Alternatively use them to make an almond milk drink. Blend them with a glass of warm milk, 5ml/ 1 tsp fructose, a pinch of nutmeg and a pinch of saffron.

DATES

Soak ten dates in ghee (a special form of clarified butter) with 1.5ml/¼ tsp of cardamon and a pinch of saffron. Cover and leave in a warm place for 2 weeks. Eat one date a day each morning; they taste delicious and will help with sexual debility and chronic fatigue.

ONIONS AND GINGER

Take 15ml/1 tbsp onion juice with 5ml/1 tsp of fresh ginger juice twice a day.

GARLIC MILK

Mix 250ml/8fl oz/1 cup milk, 50ml/ 2fl oz/¼ cup water and 1 chopped garlic clove. Boil to reduce the mixture. Drink at bedtime.

HERBAL TREATMENTS

Ayurvedic herbs to combat low libido include shatavari, ashwagandha, vidari, nutmeg and tagar.
For men Mix 5ml/1 tsp ashwagandha and 2.5ml/½ tsp vidari in a cup of warm milk and drink just before bedtime.
For women Substitute the ashwagandha with shatavari.

▼ TRY EATING THREE FIGS WITH 5ML/1 TSP OF HONEY AFTER BREAKFAST.

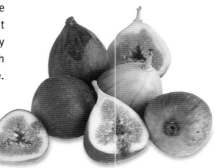

Headaches

This common problem occurs for many reasons; headaches may be stress related, caused by diet or be related to infections, poor eyesight or bad posture. Ayurveda classifies headaches into vata, pitta and kapha type.

Throbbing vata-type headaches are caused by tension and anxiety. Ease muscle tension by massaging the neck and shoulders with sesame oil; rubbing sesame oil on the top of the head and on the soles of the feet at bedtime is also said to control vata. Ayurvedic herbs to include in your diet are triphala to clear any congestion, jatamansi, brahmi and calamus.

Pitta headaches are associated with heat or burning sensations, flushed skin and visual sensitivity to light. They can be brought on by eating spicy food and by anger or frustration. A pitta headache may clear up if you eat something sweet; try some fruit. Cooling aloe vera juice can help: take 30ml/ 2 tbsp up to three times a day.

Kapha headaches are congested, dull and heavy, and often associated with sinus pain. Fresh air and plenty of exercise will help to alleviate congestion.

▼ IF YOU HAVE A HEADACHE, YOUR BLOOD SUGAR MAY BE LOW. COUNTER THIS WITH NATURAL SUGARS: A GLASS OF FRESHLY SQUEEZED FRUIT JUICE IS AN EXCELLENT CURE.

▼ IF YOU SUFFER FROM FREQUENT HEADACHES, YOUR DIET MAY BE THE CAUSE OF YOUR DISCOMFORT. KEEP A RECORD TO SEE IF ANY FOODS TRIGGER YOUR HEADACHES.

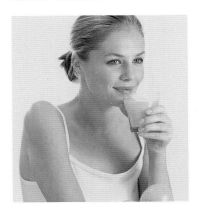

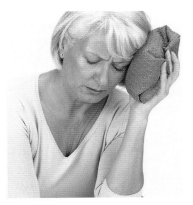

Insomnia

People in the West are likely to have a problem with excess vata as it relates to overactivity in the nervous system and leads to stress-related disorders. Insomnia is caused by an increase of vata in the mind.

Any vata-increasing influence can contribute to insomnia, including lots of travel, stress, an erratic lifestyle and the use of stimulants such as tea or coffee. Ayurvedic herbal treatment is with brahmi, jatamansi, ashwagandha and nutmeg. A foot massage with brahmi oil last thing at night may help.

Out-of-balance pitta can also contribute to insomnia when it is brought on by anger, jealousy, frustration, fever, or excess sun or heat. Herbs to include in your diet are brahmi, jatamansi, bhringaraj, shatavari and aloe vera juice. Massage brahmi oil into the head and feet.

INSOMNIA TREATMENT
As an aid to a good night's sleep, add 10ml/2 tsp fruit sugar and 2 pinches of grated nutmeg to a glass of tomato juice. Drink it late in the afternoon (16.00–17.00 hours) and follow it with an early dinner (18.00–19.00 hours).

▼ TEA, COFFEE, CHOCOLATE AND COLA CONTAIN CAFFEINE, WHICH KEEPS YOU AWAKE.

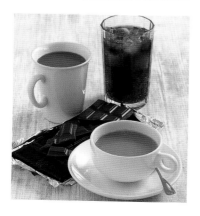

▼ SPEND TIME RELAXING BEFORE YOU PREPARE FOR BED. YOU COULD SCENT THE ROOM WITH SOOTHING ESSENTIAL OILS.

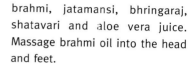

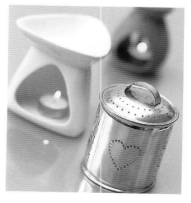

Colds and flu

The cold damp months of winter and early spring are the times of year when many people will get a cold. Symptoms typically include excess mucus production and feverishness, alternately feeling chilly or burning hot.

Kapha colds are thick and mucusy, with a heavy feeling in the head and/or body. Follow the kapha eating plan and eliminate dairy, nuts and heavy, oily food from the diet. Drink hot lemon spiced with ginger, cinnamon and cloves or cardamon, and use steam inhalations to help clear the sinuses.

The early stage of a cold is often marked by a dry, sore throat. Dryness in the body is a symptom of vata imbalance; helpful herbs include ginger, cumin, pippali, tulsi, cloves, peppermint, shatavari and ashwagandha.

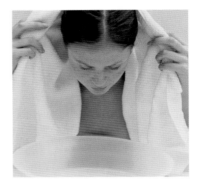

▲ A STEAM INHALATION, MADE USING GINGER ADDED TO A BOWL OF HOT WATER, HELPS RELIEVE A COLD.

When there is fever, a pitta imbalance may be indicated. Avoid hot, spicy food and use cooling herbal preparations; peppermint, spearmint, sandalwood, chrysanthemum and tulsi are all suitable.

GINGER
The best remedy for colds is ginger. It can be eaten raw, steeped in hot water and made into drinks. Its warming properties will invigorate the body and help with the elimination of toxins.

▼ MOST PEOPLE GET COLDS IN WINTER DURING THE KAPHA PHASE OF THE YEAR.

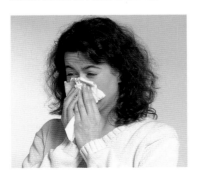

Coughs

Coughs are usually a by-product of colds and other respiratory infections. They fall into two broad categories: those that are dry and irritating, and those that are "wet" and congesting. Inflammation may be present in either type.

Vata coughs are dry and irritating with very little mucus. They may be accompanied by a dry mouth and sore throat. Herbs and spices include licorice (contra-indicated if you suffer hypertension), shatavari, ashwagandha and cardamon. A ripe banana mashed up with 5ml/1 tsp honey and a couple of pinches of black pepper is also effective; eat it two or three times a day.

Pitta coughs are usually associated with a lot of phlegm, which tends to stick on the chest. Fever or heat, combined with a burning sensation in the chest or throat may also be present. The best herbs for pitta coughs include peppermint, tulsi and sandalwood.

Kapha coughs are generally loose and productive. Keep warm and avoid damp, cold environments. A simple and effective treatment is to mix 2.5ml/½ tsp of black pepper with 5ml/1 tsp of honey and eat it on a full stomach. The heat of the black pepper will warm the body and help to drive out the cough. Ginger, lemons and cloves are also useful.

▼ TREAT A COUGH ACCORDING TO YOUR DOSHA TYPE.

▼ MAKE A WARMING LEMON DRINK TO SOOTHE A DRY COUGH.

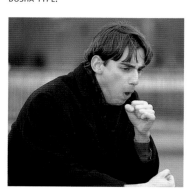

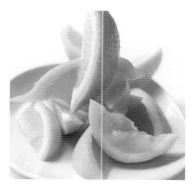

Urinary infections

Cystitis is one of the most common infections of the urinary tract, particularly in women. It is generally a bacterial infection and should always be treated straight away because of the risk of it spreading to the kidneys.

Cystitis is mainly a pitta condition because it burns and is inflamed and hot. Avoid hot foods and spices and use plenty of coriander (cilantro). Other remedies include aloe vera juice (contra-indicated in

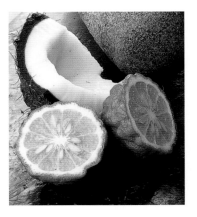

▲ Coconut and lime are recommended for pitta cystitis.

Tips for treating cystitis

- Avoid tea, coffee and alcoholic drinks.
- Personal hygiene is extremely important; always pull the toilet paper up and away from the body after defecation.
- Bathe with unperfumed oils and soaps until the infection has cleared.
- Coriander (cilantro), cumin and fennel tea is a good tonic. Use 1.5ml/¼ tsp of each herb per cup of boiling water.

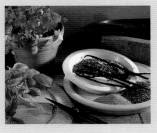

pregnancy), lime juice, coconut, pomegranate and sandalwood.

Kapha-type cystitis is accompanied by congestion and mucus in the urinary tract; the urine is often pale or clear. The treatments are cinnamon, trikatu combined with shilajit, gokshura and gokshuradi guggulu. Avoid salt, sugar and all dairy products.

In vata people, cystitis will tend to be less intense. Herbal remedies you can try include shilajit with bala, ashwagandha and shatavari.

Skin problems

A glowing complexion and silky, "baby-soft" skin is a reality that many of us only dream about. Skin problems are extremely common and can range in severity from the occasional spot to chronic conditions such as psoriasis.

Vata skin problems will be dry and rough and include chapped lips, cracked heels, "sandpaper" hands and dandruff. Avoid letting the skin dry out and exposing it to cold and/or windy weather. Herbal remedies for vata skin are triphala and satisabgol (the latter is useful if you are also constipated).

Excess pitta causes skin problems that itch, burn or erupt into spots or rashes. The skin is usually red, swollen, raised or inflamed, often with a yellow head or pus discharge. Avoid sun, heat, hot baths or saunas, and increase your

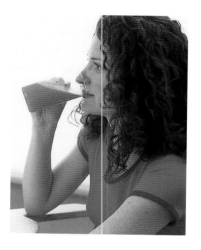

▲ JUICES ARE GOOD FOR THE SKIN. DRINK THEM WHEN THEY ARE FRESHLY MADE.

intake of water, salads, raw vegetables and fruits. Cooling spices are turmeric, coriander and saffron. Skincare products made with the fruit and seeds of the Neem tree are also useful.

Greasy, oily skin indicates a kapha imbalance. Increase your exercise and follow the kapha eating plan. Useful herbs include calamus, cinnamon, cloves, dry ginger, trikatu formula and turmeric.

TIPS FOR BEAUTIFUL SKIN

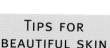

- Begin the day with a glass of hot water containing a squeeze of lemon.
- Take a daily capsule of turmeric.
- Enjoy regular massage.
- Use Neem or sandalwood soap for bathing.
- For some natural colour, drink fresh carrot juice and eat cooked beetroot (beet).

Face and body cleansers

The very simplest cleansers consist of little more than puréed fruits. Face or body masks can be made from these blends with the simple addition of oatmeal or besan (chickpea or gram flour) to these ingredients.

Choose ripe fruits and vegetables to make a nourishing facepack. You can get away with simply squashing softer fruits, although harder types will need grating or puréeing. Experiment to find what has the best result on your skin.

▶ IF YOU HAVE VERY SENSITIVE SKIN, AVOID GRAPE AND SHARP-TASTING CITRUS FRUITS, OR MODIFY BY COMBINING WITH BANANA.

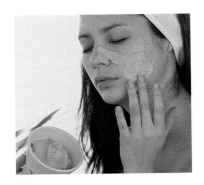

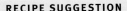

RECIPE SUGGESTION

SKIN REJUVENATOR
This is kind to mature skin and can help reduce the appearance of wrinkles.
INGREDIENTS
handful of fresh scented geranium (Pelargonium graveolens) leaves
rose water to cover

Soak the geranium leaves in rose water for a few hours until softened, then spread on your face and lie down for 15–30 minutes. Rinse with cool water.

RECIPE SUGGESTION

AVOCADO FACEPACK
A mix of egg white and lemon juice suits oily complexions, but the addition of avocado, rich in natural oils, makes this a great soother for dry skin too.
INGREDIENTS
1 avocado
5 ml/1 tsp lemon juice
1 egg white

Mash the avocado, mix in the other ingredients and apply to the face. Leave for up to 20 minutes, then rinse with cool water.

Body cleansers

Exfoliating the body should form a regular part of any skincare routine. Gritty ingredients like clay, oatmeal and besan (chickpea or gram flour) help to draw out dirt from deep in the pores. Oat flour is very soothing for eczema, while chickpea flour can leave the skin feeling taut, so is best combined with other dry ingredients.

Mix the mask to a thick, gritty consistency that won't slide straight off the skin when applied. As with all face and body masks, experiment on the back of your hand first before beginning a full-body treatment. Leave the mask for up to 20 minutes before massaging away and rinsing with warm water.

▼ Treat your whole body to a revitaliz-ing mask that sloughs off dead cells, letting skin shine.

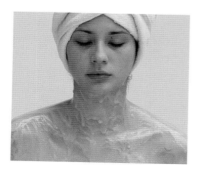

Hair care

Shining, lustrous hair is a beauty available to most women. Herbal applications can be prepared to target everything from an itchy scalp to heat-damaged tresses. Many of these plant-based remedies also have wonderful scents.

Traditionally, people massaged their hair with oil to keep it healthy and to counteract the drying effects of heat. Fragments of a dried tree resin called sambraani would be burned and the hair allowed to dry in its fragrant smoke after washing. Harsh shampoos and chemical treatments were unknown. Despite the range of hair products now available, many people are turning

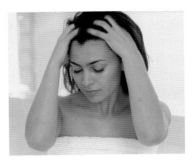

▲ Use your fingers to comb the mixture through your hair down to the tips before rinsing out.

Tips to combat scalp problems

These blends can be made in a screwtop glass jar and shaken to mix before using. Work into the scalp and leave overnight if possible; if not, a minimum of three hours is essential.
•To combat dandruff, try 5ml/ 1 tsp each of castor oil, mustard oil and coconut oil. If your scalp is not too sensitive, combine 1 part lemon juice to 2 parts coconut oil.
• To soothe an itchy scalp, grind some dried jasmine root into a bowl of lime juice. Massage into damp hair, then rinse thoroughly.

back to tried and tested formulas, some of which blend traditional knowledge with modern convenience. Instead of crushing leaves from the neem tree to enhance the condition of your hair, for example, you can now pick up a bottle of neem shampoo or conditioner.

Hair and scalp problems may suggest a dosha imbalance, though they may also be aggravated by the effects of stress, harsh shampoos, excessive heating or exposure to air conditioning. A dry and flaky scalp is often caused by the drying effect of aggravated vata dosha.

WHAT IS YOUR HAIR TYPE?

Like the rest of our bodies, our hair can show signs of our predominant doshas. If your constitution is mainly vata, you're likely to have dark, dry, coarse or frizzy hair that's prone to tangling, split ends and dandruff.

Pittas are often blondes or redheads. They have enviable hair – fine and silky – but it needs looking after to prevent a tendency to go thin and grey before its time. It tends to be oily, but harsh shampoos make matters worse and can accelerate aging.

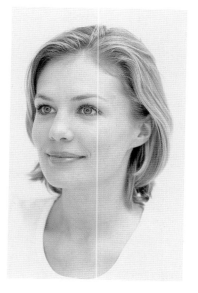

▲ PITTA HAIR REWARDS GENTLE TREATMENT WITH SILKY SLEEKNESS. DON'T BE TEMPTED TO USE HARSH PRODUCTS THAT MAY CAUSE THINNING. AN IMBALANCE OF PITTA IS THE COMMONEST CAUSE OF HAIR PROBLEMS.

TIPS FOR ADDING SHINE

- Lemon or lime is a staple of home-made hair treatments. Combine the juice of ½ a lemon or one lime with two cups of warm water, or use rose water for one half of this amount, and use as a rinse after shampooing and conditioning.
- For dry hair, massage a beaten egg into the hair after washing and rinsing.
- To treat heat-damaged hair, combine an egg with 30ml/2 tbsp castor oil, 5ml/1 tsp cider vinegar or wine vinegar and 5ml/1 tsp glycerine. Massage into the hair and leave as long as you like before rinsing off.

People of kapha constitution may complain about their oiliness, but they have the least to worry about with hair that's naturally thick, glossy and wavy.

If suffering continually dull hair or an inflamed scalp, an Ayurvedic practitioner may suggest changes to the diet, including more green leafy vegetables, salads, milk, fruits and sprouts, buttermilk, yeast, wheat germ, soy beans and grains.

Index

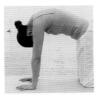

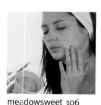